MW01137360

Lipid

LUNACY

Diet delusions
and what really
causes heart disease

Editors
Prof. Paul J Rosch
Prof. Abdullah A Alabdulgader

Published by Columbus Publishing Ltd 2020
www.columbuspublishing.co.uk

ISBN 978-1-907797-736
Rev 20200706

Copyright © 2020 individual authors

Each contributing author has asserted their right to be identified as the authors of their work in accordance with the Copyright, Designs and Patents Act 1988.

All rights reserved. No part of this publication may be reproduced, stored in a retrieval system, or transmitted in any form or by any means, electronic, mechanical, photocopying or otherwise without the prior permission of the respective author.

Cover design by Andy Harcombe

Typesetting by Raffaele Bolelli Gallevi

Brand and product names are trademarks or registered trademarks of their respective owners.

The information provided in this book should not be construed as personal medical advice or instruction. No action should be taken based solely on the contents of this book. Readers should consult appropriate health professionals on any matter relating to their health and well-being.

The information and opinions provided here are believed to be accurate and sound and are based on the best judgments of the authors, but readers who fail to consult appropriate health authorities assume the risk of any injuries. Neither the authors nor the publisher can be held responsible or liable for any loss or claim arising from the use, or misuse, of the content of this book.

COLUMBUS PUBLISHING

Dedication to Editor Professor Paul Rosch

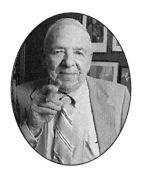

Prof. Paul Rosch

Dr Paul J. Rosch, born June 30, 1927, sadly passed away on Wednesday, February 26, 2020, after complications from a fall. He was 92 years old. He never got to see the final version of this book, but his contribution to its inception and his drive to get it completed was paramount in getting the work to press.

Dr Rosch MA, MD, FACP was Chairman of the Board of The American Institute of Stress, Clinical Professor of Medicine and Psychiatry at New York Medical College, and Honorary Vice President of the International Stress Management Association. He completed his internship and residency training at Johns Hopkins Hospital and subsequently at the Walter Reed Army Hospital and Institute of Research, where he was Director of the Endocrine Section.

Dr Rosch was the recipient of many honors, at home and abroad, including the New York State Medical Society's Outstanding Physician's Award, the Schering Award, the American Rural Health Association's International Distinguished Service Award, the Innovation Award of The International Society for the Study of Subtle Energies and Energy Medicine, and The I.M. Sechenov Memorial Medal from The Russian Academy of Medical Sciences.

Dr Rosch was a Fellow and Life Member of The American College of Physicians and served as President of the New York State Society of Internal Medicine, President of the Pavlovian Society and Expert

Consultant on Stress to the United States Centers for Disease Control. He was also Chairman of the International Foundation for Biopsychosocial Development and Human Health. He was a member of the Board of Governors of The American Academy of Experts in Traumatic Stress, Scientific Advisory Council of the Alzheimer's Prevention Foundation, and Clinical Professor of Medicine in Psychiatry at the University of Maryland School of Medicine. He was editor-in-chief of *Stress Medicine*, published by John Wiley & Sons, Inc. in the U.K., and was on the editorial board of several relevant journals.

In addition to these accomplishments, Dr Rosch was a member of the International Network of Cholesterol Skeptics (THINCS) and a fearless critic of the diet-heart hypothesis. He shared his views on this topic during an appearance as a speaker at the first of CrossFit Health's lecture series, known colloquially as the "Derelict Doctors Club," in 2018. He was always generous with his time and intellect, up until the end of his life.

In his editor's introduction to *Fat and Cholesterol Don't Cause Heart Attacks and Statins Are not the Solution*, a seminal collection of scientific critiques of the diet-heart hypothesis and the poor research upon which the fat and cholesterol scare was built, Dr Rosch wrote:

If you ask anyone "What causes heart attacks", the vast majority, including physicians, would undoubtedly blame high cholesterol from eating too much fat, or include this along with unavoidable influences like heredity and stress. That's not surprising, since this dietary fat ⇨ elevated cholesterol ⇨ heart attacks scenario has been repeated over and over so many times for the past 70 years, that it has become accepted as gospel. ... reducing fat intake, especially saturated fat, has been U.S. policy for the past 35 years. These official guidelines are the basis for determining the foods that will be used in the military, government cafeterias, schools, food assistance programs, industry food formulations, and restaurant recipes, as well as recommendations made by nutritionists and dieticians. And since they were also endorsed by leading authorities and prestigious organizations such as the American Heart Association and the American College of Cardiology, it was assumed that restricting fats would provide cardioprotective and other health benefits. The advent of statins, which allegedly prevented heart disease by lowering cholesterol, appeared to prove the validity of the lipid hypothesis, and statins quickly became the best-selling prescription drugs ever. ...

The tragedy is that none of these low cholesterol low fat recommendations had any scientific support. ... The sad fact is that this low fat diet should never have been introduced, and the consequences of this error have been disastrous. Only 15% of the population was obese when the low-fat guidelines appeared in 1980. This has now increased to 35% in adults, and 17% in children and teenagers. If obesity rates continue on their current trajectories, 50% or more adults could be obese by 2030. And the diet heart idea has even had more catastrophic results.

A recent study of physically active healthy people who took statins for 90 to 365 days reported that their risk of developing diabetes and diabetic complications doubled over the next five years compared to controls. Short term statin use was not associated with any decrease in cardiovascular events, so for healthy people in particular, statins can do more harm than good, especially since type 2 diabetes is a significant risk factor for heart disease. It would appear that the lipid hypothesis will continue to persist and prevail as long as it remains profitable for statin and low-fat food manufacturers and other vested interests.

It is for this clear and bold resolution to objectively follow the scientific evidence wherever it might lead, despite the naysaying of industry forces or popular understanding, that Dr Rosch will be long remembered by CrossFit, Inc. and its intellectual associates.

Greg Glassman observes:

The CrossFit nutrition prescription has stood in opposition to the high-carb, low-fat mainstream orthodoxy for decades. Until recently, our position was rather detached from the world of academia, governmental guidelines, and industry. In the independent course of our daily business — physical fitness training — we came to the clinical understanding that high consumption of refined carbohydrate retards fitness and degrades health while fats and proteins have the opposite effect. Millions of CrossFit practitioners have observed and benefited from this knowledge in 15,000 CrossFit affiliates around the world. ...

The first edition of Fat and Cholesterol Don't Cause Heart Attacks was a revelation to us — not because it inspired reforms to our prescription, but because it laid out in damning and forensic detail the verification of our skepticism. That book's elucidation of the lengths taken to advance and preserve the profitable notion of cholesterol's deadly effects has become a fundamental contribution to our understanding of the ills of modern medicine and the abuse of the public's trust in "science."

Long-time friends and colleagues of Dr Rosch remember him accordingly:

At the age of collective wisdom, in 2008 Paul Rosch's scientific blessings extended to the eastern hemisphere. I invited him first to co-organize the King of Organs 2008 conference. I was captured with his sharp mind and comprehensive knowledge. He was cofounder and deputy president of the unique cardiac conference, King of Organs for Advanced Cardiac Sciences, for four consecutive conferences: 2008, 2010, 2012 and 2019. He energised me with his marvellous spirit. His extraordinary scientific character created scientific revolutions in the metabolic arena, disclosing the cholesterol myth and homocysteine metabolism as well as the heart mind sciences and stress management. I admired him as my spiritual father and mutually he was founding himself in my spirit when he was at my age. In February 26, 2020, Paul's soul responded to the heavens' call. At personal level, I lost a father, friend and life model. Paul's footsteps, bravery and wisdom in life will remain a shining star for all generations.
God Bless his magnificent soul.

Prof. Abdullah Alabdulgader

Paul was a great man, and not many people can lay claim to that word. He was extraordinarily intelligent, and he used that intelligence wisely — to question things that didn't make sense. That led him into the world of cholesterol and heart disease, while he would have been even better known by others for his significant contributions to the fields of psychiatry and stress. He had breadth and depth in knowledge and never lost interest in soaking up more. He was driven and hard-working, and he never let anything slip, but it was his sharpness that really impressed. He was razor sharp, an attribute that would manifest itself in wit or insight. Either way, it made him informative and fun to be around. He will be much missed by family, friends, colleagues, and entire academic movements.

Zoë Harcombe

With Paul's passing the world has lost a brilliant scientist, a great man, my friend & mentor. Paul demanded integrity and accuracy in science. He had no tolerance for the deception underlying the demonization of cholesterol and the peddling of statins to the masses.

I was close with Paul for almost a decade. I was honored to be a co-author with him on our joint publications on heart disease and cholesterol.

I had the pleasure to be with him at our first conference together in Saudi Arabia in 2012. I'll never forget when a cardiologist/speaker at that meeting was promoting statin effectiveness using inflated relative risk values. Paul stood up and pointed his finger at the speaker and said with such great force – you are deceiving these people! You are leading them to believe statins have great benefits, when in fact statins are harmful and their benefits are meager. The speaker and crowd were taken aback by this small elderly man who spoke with such authority.

I'm glad I was able to make a tribute to him at a CrossFit talk I gave in 2018. I cherished our time together, he inspired me and he helped me to be a better scientist. Paul has left a legacy for others to follow in his footsteps, to promote integrity in all aspects of scientific inquiry.

David Diamond

I consider it a great privilege to have met and worked with Paul. Even at his youthful age of 92, he could fill a large room with energy. Always polite, thoughtful, witty, and very bright, Paul had fascinating insights on any topic that you'd like to talk about with him. He was blessed with one of the sharpest minds, and he used that gift to challenge conventional wisdom and move science forward in a positive way. He made great contributions in all areas that he decided to have an interest in, and he will be missed, of course, by his family and friends, but also by everyone who was fortunate enough to have met him.

Andy Harcombe

There are many people that I have "met" on the Internet but sadly never had the chance to meet in person, but I always admire those who stick doggedly to the task of scientific truth and honesty even in the face of *denigration and vilification. Those who swim against the tide will always struggle, and Paul was in one sense a modern Galileo. His wisdom will be greatly missed but those who remain must continue his work.*

Andrew Bamji

Paul Rosch was a true pioneer in the arena of rational evaluation of the lipid hypothesis. And like many true pioneers, he took a few arrows in the back, but he persevered. Despite antagonism and attacks from those who stood to profit from chimera of LDL reduction at all cost, he continued to fight and publish till the end. With his passing, science has lost a voice for truth and transparency, a voice that will be much missed by those who seek to restore the integrity of scientific inquiry.

Michael Eades

Paul Rosch was one of the greatest mentors and inspirators I had in medical science. He was also a true friend. Apart from this he gave support and help to some of my ideas which resulted in different studies and researches. He has been my co-author in the two latest studies. I owe to Paul all the opportunities for disclosure and also the scientific reach that, eventually, I might get in the future.

Carlos Monteiro

Paul was a man or rare qualities. A seeker of the truth, unafraid to look at new ideas, brave enough to challenge the status quo. Some people see the waves, and learn to surf on them, to the adulation of crowds. Others are far more interested in finding out where the waves come from – and learn to make their own. Paul was one such. A maker of waves. I am glad that I came to know him.

Malcolm Kendrick

About the Editor Professor Abdullah Alabdulgader

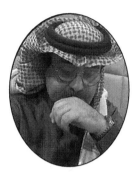

Prof. Abdullah Abdulrhman Alabdulgader

Professor Abdullah Alabdulgader, MD, DCH(I), DCH(Edinb), MRCP(UK), ABP, FRCP(UK) was born in Al-Khobar and raised in Al-Hasa, in the eastern part of Saudi Arabia. Al-Hasa is in the middle of ancient wisdom with cultural and religious sobriety, while being embraced in marvellous harmony with the gigantic oil industry. His genetic lineage extends to the Al-Ansar tribe where, over 40 generations ago, Abu Ayub Alansari was one of the elite partners of prophet Muhammad.

Professor Alabdulgader graduated from the college of medicine and medical sciences, King Faisal University, in 1991. Immediately, after graduation, he was involved in extensive medical training, cascaded at different levels of specialties, until 1997 where he was certified with five medical degrees. This qualified him to double major specialty in paediatrics and adolescent medicine and subspecialty in paediatric cardiology with awards from Saudi Arabia, Ireland and the United Kingdom.

He excelled to achieve a record achievement in becoming a member of the Royal Colleges of Physicians (UK), having completed all examinations and requirements in just 12 months and becoming an MRCP(UK) holder at the age of 27. Soon afterward he established the first foundation for congenital heart services in eastern Saudi Arabia.

In addition to optimizing the organization of clinical services, research was one of his paramount priorities. Professor Alabdulgader has long been fascinated by the epidemiology of cardiac dysmorphology in humans. He initiated examination of the incidence and demographic characteristics for congenital heart disease for the first time in his part of the world. This scientific step heralded the onset of one of the major scientific projects in human history – concerned with discovering the environmental and genetic risk factors of congenital heart diseases in an attempt to discover the mysterious secrets of human heart dysmorphogenesis, with the ultimate aim of overcoming the disease in human species.

In 2001, Professor Alabdulgader was granted a special governmental scholarship to further sub-specialize in cardiac electrophysiology and electrical rhythm devices. This study was undertaken in Edmonton, Alberta, Canada. During this time, he was able to describe, for the first time in medical literature, unique congenital anomalies, in native Canadian new-borns, from Calgary University hospital.

He is well known for founding the Prince Sultan Cardiac Center, in Al-Hasa, Saudi Arabia (PSCCH) after a generous donation from the late crown prince of the country HRH Prince Sultan bin Abdulaziz. PSCCH, today, is one of the leading tertiary care cardiac centers in the middle east and the world.

Professor Alabdulgader's holistic universal scope in science and the universe led him to establish the reputable King of Organs Congress for Advanced Cardiac Sciences, where the wisdom dictates perceiving the human heart as a souvenir of the soul and a cradle of the mind and wisdom, with extensive and delicate symphony resonating to higher energetic levels of collective consciousness. Critical conceptual faith and reasoning behind the King of Organs establishment was to rescue humanity from the historical myths with absent scientific insight, such as the great cholesterol myth.

Professor Alabdulgader, as the congress founder and president, and the late professor Paul Rosch, as his congress deputy, devoted a full day of scientific debate to expose the cholesterol myth in four consecutive international conferences (2008, 2010, 2012 and 2019). This book represents the fourth day lectures from the 2019 congress.

In other work, Professor Alabdulgader collaborated with HeartMath Institute, California, USA, where he was able to establish a special detection system to record the planetary Schumann frequencies. He was awarded the world gold medal from WOSCO (Great Britain-2012) for establishing unique direction in astrobiology and cardiac sciences exploring the human heart rate variability orchestration with Schumann resonances and solar winds. In the same year he was awarded the Diploma of honour from the International Committee on geological and environmental change (GEOCHANGE), Munich, Germany.

In 2018, he led a scientific team from HeartMath Institute, NASA, along with a reputable European scientist, in the longest human record synchronizing human heart rate variability with Schumann resonances, solar winds and cosmic rays. This achievement was published in Nature scientific reports in February 2018.

Nowadays, Professor Alabdulgader is leading a number of international projects concerned with investigating the role of the very low frequency band of the heart rate variability in inflammation and systemic hypertension to treat systemic hypertension without medications. The Saudi Homocysteine Atherosclerosis and Cancer Trial (SAHACT) utilizes cellular pathways with simple nutrients to combat atherosclerosis and cancer in human, and other projects. In the clinical arena he is a senior interventional congenital cardiologist and electrophysiologist performing ablation interventions with radiofrequency as well as cryoablation technologies utilizing cardiac electrical mapping to cure cardiac arrhythmias.

Professor Alabdulgader is a scientific board member and editorial board member of many international organizations and journals in the USA, UK, Germany, Switzerland, China, India and other countries. He has received many acknowledging letters and honouring events and gifts from King Salman, Princes, and world authorities. At the moment, he is the senior scientist and chief physician in PSCCH and the leader of the research and biostatistics services, preparing for the next King of Organs congress with higher consciousness for the better future of humankind.

Contents

Part One

Introduction and Background

Introduction
How and Why This Book Was Assembled
Paul J. Rosch, MD

This book is based on presentations by THINCS members (The International Network of Cholesterol Sceptics), which I arranged for the fifth International Congress for Advanced Cardiac Sciences in Saudi Arabia in March 2019, as I had done for these previous "King of Organs" conferences. In some respects, it is a sequel to *Fat and Cholesterol Don't Cause Heart Attacks – And Statins Are Not The Solution*, since it provides further insights to those chapters by many of the current authors. The *Fat and Cholesterol* book was dedicated to Dr Uffe Ravnskov, the founder and still leader of THINCS. This book is dedicated to Abdullah Alabdulgader, Consultant to the Prince Sultan Cardiac Center, who sponsors these events, and to Greg Glassman, Founder of CrossFit, for this organization's support of THINCS.

Although Greg Glassman, did not participate in this event, he has contributed the following magnificent Foreword, which explains how the millions of CrossFit practitioners in 15,000 CrossFit affiliates around the world have benefited from learning that sugar and refined carbohydrates, rather than cholesterol or LDL, are the real culprits in coronary heart disease. It is a scholarly paean of praise for Uffe Ravnskov and other THINCS members who have been persecuted professionally and personally for criticizing the hypothesis that saturated fat → elevated cholesterol → coronary heart disease. It also explains how this fallacious doctrine has been perpetrated by powerful food, beverage, and drug companies that fund research favorable to their interests.

His Foreword is followed by Abdullah Alabdulgader's Presidential Welcome outlining the purpose of this Congress and Uffe Ravnskov's Keynote Address on why THINCS was created in 2003 and how it has evolved since then. The remaining chapters fall under the following three headings:

What Does the Future Hold?

Despite all the numerous bona fide criticisms presented here and previously, the cholesterol juggernaut rolls on. It is fuelled by the desire to preserve and increase huge profits, rather than improve health, as illustrated by the current frenzy to develop CETP (Cholesteryl ester transfer protein) and PCSK9 (Proprotein convertase subtilisin/kexin type 9) inhibitors to lower cholesterol and LDL as much as possible. This is based on the same old but erroneous assumption that LDL causes coronary atherosclerosis, regardless of overwhelming contrary evidence. The futility of this approach also applies to the use of siRNA molecules to inhibit PCSK9 by a different mechanism that requires an injection twice a year.

The current situation is likely to persist because of the powerful cholesterol cartel of Big Pharma, low fat food manufacturers and testing equipment companies that have gained control over regulatory agencies, the media, prominent organizations, academia, and authorities, who are the recipients of their lavish largesse. In addition, as Max Planck warned, *"A new scientific truth does not triumph by convincing its opponents and making them see the light, but rather because its opponents eventually die and a new generation grows up that is familiar with it."* And Arthur Schopenhauer noted, *"All truth passes through three stages. First, it is ridiculed, second it is violently opposed, and Third, it is accepted as self-evident."*

Claude Bernard emphasized that good health and life itself depends on preserving the stability of the *milieu intérieur* (internal environment) whenever it is threatened, which Walter Cannon referred to as homeostasis. This means the ability to automatically and instantly maintain blood pressure, heart rate and blood concentrations of oxygen, glucose, sodium, potassium and other vital constituents within fairly rigid limits. But how does communication take place in the body? The role of the central nervous system with its antagonistic but complementary sympathetic and parasympathetic components is fairly well delineated. The endocrine system has its own balancing mechanisms in which the secretion of hormones is regulated by feedback from target glands or metabolic consequences. Much less is known about how equilibrium is maintained in neurotransmitter networks or in the immune system, which has both hardwired and humoral nervous system connections. In addition, our current concept of how communication takes place in the body is at a chemical/molecular level as we visualize small peptide messengers fitting into specific receptor sites on cell walls, much like keys that fit into certain keyhole sites on cell walls. Such physical structural matching, which could occur only on a random-collision basis, does not explain the myriad instantaneous and constantly changing reactions that occur in "fight or flight" responses to severe stress.

There is an emerging paradigm of communication at a physical/ atomic level that may not only provide some answers, but also insights into widely acknowledged but poorly understood phenomena such as the placebo effect, the power of prayer and a firm faith, as well as the benefits of therapeutic touch, and acupuncture. EEG waves may not merely reflect the noise of the machinery of the brain, but signals being sent to specific sites on cell walls. The heart's electrical field is over 100 times greater than the brain's, its magnetic field is 5,000 times more powerful, can be detected up to 3 feet away from the body, and can influence the EEG of someone with whom you are in close physical contact. As with neuropeptide stimulation, these emanations may stimulate specific receptors on cell walls to send energy signals to the interior of the cell to activate various enzyme systems or to replicate itself. Thus, in addition to being a protective shield, the cell wall can act as a powerful amplifier for subtle electromagnetic forces. All communication in the body ultimately takes place at a physical/ atomic level via subtle electromagnetic signals.

As Lord Kelvin warned, "*To measure is to know*," and "*If you can't measure it, you can't improve it.*" That certainly applies to stress, and HRV (heart rate variability), the subtle beat to beat variation in heart rate, is probably the most accurate objective method of measuring stress. Diminished HRV is a powerful predictor of sudden death and recent refinements now allow the ability to not only measure HRV in real time, but to restore dangerous levels to normal. Physicians in the future will be prescribing frequencies rather than pills, radiation and surgery. This has already taken place with respect to the treatment of cancer, diverse neuropsychiatric disorders, stress related complaints, and job stress, because it is much safer and more effective, as demonstrated below. (References 1-7)

Paul J. Rosch, MD

References

1. Pasche B, Jiminez H, Zimmerman J, Pennison M, *et al.* Systemic Treatment of Cancer With Low and Safe Levels of Radiofrequency Electromagnetic Fields Amplitude-Modulated at Tumor-Specific Frequencies, pp. 299-306 in Rosch PJ ed. Bioelectric and Subtle Energy Medicine. 2nd edition. CRC Press (Taylor & Frances Group) 2015; Boca Raton.

2. White PJ, Jolesz FA. MRI-Guided Focused Ultrasound. A Method for Noninvasive Surgery and Other Clinical Applications, pp. 363-374 in Rosch PJ ed. Bioelectric and Subtle Energy Medicine. 2nd edition. CRC Press (Taylor & Frances Group) 2015; Boca Raton.

3. George MS, Short EB, Kerns S, Xingbao L *et al.* Repetitive Magnetic Stimulation for Depression and Other Indications, pp. 169-188 in Rosch PJ ed. Bioelectric and Subtle Energy Medicine. 2nd edition. CRC Press (Taylor & Frances Group) 2015; Boca Raton.

4. Roth Y, Zangen A. Noninvasive Deep TMS Therapy for Diverse Neuropsychiatric Disorders, pp. 227-253 in Rosch PJ ed. Bioelectric and Subtle Energy Medicine. 2nd edition. CRC Press (Taylor & Frances Group) 2015; Boca Raton.

5. Kirsch DJ, Marksberry JA. The Evolution of Cranial Electrotherapy Stimulation for Anxiety, Insomnia, Depression and Pain, pp. 189-212 in Rosch PJ ed. Bioelectric and Subtle Energy Medicine. 2nd edition. CRC Press (Taylor & Frances Group) 2015; Boca Raton.

6. Zabara J. Vagus Nerve Stimulation and the Neurocybernetic Prosthesis: The Way Forward, pp. 25-266 in Rosch PJ ed. Bioelectric and Subtle Energy Medicine. 2nd edition. CRC Press (Taylor & Frances Group) 2015; Boca Raton.

7. Low A, McCraty R. Heart rate variability: New Perspectives on Assessment of Stress and Health risk at the Workplace. 2018; Heart Mind 2:16-27.

Foreword

Greg Glassman, Founder CrossFit

The CrossFit nutrition prescription has stood in opposition to the high-carb, low-fat mainstream orthodoxy for decades. Until recently, our position was rather detached from the world of academia, governmental guidelines, and industry. In the independent course of our daily business – physical fitness training – we came to the clinical understanding that high consumption of refined carbohydrate retards fitness and degrades health while fats and proteins have the opposite effect. Millions of CrossFit practitioners have observed and benefited from this knowledge in 15,000 CrossFit affiliates around the world. Mainstream dietary advice, consumed as it was with the frantic urging to reduce cholesterol at whatever cost, was irrelevant to our daily work. We posted Uffe Ravnskov's *Cholesterol Myths* to our website in 2003, recognizing that it comported with our observed reality, and went about our business. Meanwhile, the world outside the CrossFit gym grew sicker.

The first edition of *Fat and Cholesterol Don't Cause Heart Attacks* was a revelation to us – not because it inspired reforms to our prescription, but because it laid out in damning and forensic detail the verification of our skepticism. That book's elucidation of the lengths taken to advance and preserve the profitable notion of cholesterol's deadly effects has become a fundamental contribution to our understanding of the ills of modern medicine and the abuse of the public's trust in "science."

The disasters of mainstream nutrition science – specifically, in this case, the lipid hypothesis that guided millions of people toward chronic disease – are the result of corruption almost perfect in scope and reach. We use "corruption" here fully cognizant of a dual meaning: corruption in terms of the spreading stain of special interests, financial motivation, and bad actions taken for personal gain, and also corruption in the sense that a file or disk can be corrupted – damaged beyond the point of usefulness. The reality of both forms of corruption is self-evident from a look at the outcomes of nutrition and pharmaceutical science for the past several decades: declining life expectancy in industrial nations; an impending tsunami of diabetes and other chronic diseases far beyond the carrying capacity of health-care infrastructure and personnel; and industry capture of the governmental, academic, and scientific bodies entrusted with public health. The "science-backed" nutrition guidelines haven't worked. The near-universal prescription of statins and other pharmaceutical solutions hasn't worked. These panaceas and campaigns haven't worked because the predominant conception of animal fat and cholesterol as deadly drivers of heart disease and other chronic maladies is not substantiated by the scientific evidence. The foundational claims and premises have been corrupted, at a terrible cost.

Yet despite these horrific outcomes, the perverse incentive structure of the medical and nutritional sciences remains intact. The food, beverage, and pharmaceutical industries fund research favorable to their interests. The dominant journals and academies amplify and codify this research, assisted by the dubious process of peer review, a system seemingly designed to insert human error, susceptibility, and personal weakness into scientific investigation and dissemination. Nutrition reporting encourages a popular understanding influenced more by the loudest voices than the most accurate. Alternative perspectives are thus shut out of the discussion, relegated to the margins.

Where do *Lipid Lunacy* and its contributors fall in this grim landscape? What is the perspective of those whose research and scientific investigations have led them to a very different conclusion regarding diet and nutrition?

The authors who have contributed to this text are defined by two personal characteristics: They are intelligent and insightful enough to recognize the decades-spanning failures of the dominant mainstream view, and they are brave enough to declare accordingly that the emperor has no clothes. In the realm of academic science, this is a distinct kind of bravery. Every incentive encourages the scientist to fall in line. Publications, academic positions, research funding – the stock and trade, the very sustenance of an academic career

– are apportioned to those whose work and opinions substantiate the claims that are in vogue. Then there is the simple element of reputation: Few serious academics earnestly desire to be labeled a quack, a crank, a "denier." And further yet, consider the sheer gall necessary to pit oneself against the pharmaceutical industry, the food and beverage industries, and the governmental bodies that have allied themselves so closely with these powerful interests.

What does it mean, then, that these varied individuals have come together into a cohort of skeptics, into what we at CrossFit have termed "the legitosphere"? What kind of scientific and moral alternative can they provide to the orthodoxy of consensus science – an understanding that lays claim to the authority of science but is reached via popularity, path dependence, and the great motivation of going along to get along? (The science produced by way of consensus, of course, is not science at all. On the contrary, the homogeneity of opinion rigidly enforced by fear of departure from the approved mainstream perspective is absolutely damning to real innovation and discovery and thus antithetical to the pursuits of science rightly considered.)

Our authors here form a very different kind of body. While their opinions may overlap, while many of their hypotheses follow a similar trajectory, they find themselves in a similar location precisely because they were willing to stand alone. Each independently arrived at the same place of opposition to the mainstream view, driven by their own skepticism and determination to follow the truth regardless of where it led. For these reasons, their hypotheses do not toe a definitive party line. Rather, they represent the investigations of individual minds that could not accept claims incompatible with their intellectual principles and observations. Our authors are united not by adherence to dogma but by the courage of their own convictions, which defines them as much as does their scientific acumen. It is an honor to support them individually and introduce their collective work as presented here in *Lipid Lunacy*.

Greg Glassman

Founder, CrossFit, Inc.

King of Organs Presidential Address

Abdullah A. Alabdulgader, MD

It is a great pleasure and honor for the Prince Sultan Cardiac Center to welcome all of you to the Kingdom of Saudi Arabia for The Fifth International Congress for Advanced Cardiac Sciences (King of Organs 2019). This unique, magnificent scientific event is heralding the onset of our second decade of the world of King of Organs and its famous scientific theme "Heart Sciences from Genes to Galaxies." This has progressively evolved over the last four congresses to culminate in this event, which explains the global and universal role of the human heart.

We have been calling for a revolution in the practice of cardiac sciences and a recognition that the heart is not merely a pump, but a supreme master organ that controls our emotional, spiritual, and physical health. As will be demonstrated, its magnetic field, which is 5,000 times more powerful than the brain's, can interact and influence others in close proximity, as well as geomagnetic and solar forces. Another top priority of this event will be exploring the role of cellular pathways in the pathogenesis of cardiovascular disease, especially with respect to the unappreciated role of homocysteine. This will be discussed in a presentation dealing with the SAHACT (Saudi Arabian Homocysteine Atherosclerosis And Cancer Trial) that is now underway to prevent these and other deadly diseases. In addition, we will update our progress in the genetic and environmental risk factors in congenital heart disease project that is also being conducted under the aegis of the Prince Sultan Cardiac Center. We will devote the final day to a discussion of advances in the diagnosis and treatment of coronary heart disease, novel theories about its cause, such as the role of inflammation and coagulation, and the consequences of such efforts. There will be six parallel workshops to provide more information and hands on experience for specific topics. These cutting edge and state of the art presentations will not be a repetition or regurgitation of current conventional thinking or entrenched dogma, since, as the Nobel Laureate Richard Feynman noted:

"I would rather have questions that can't be answered than answers that can't be questioned" and *"I learned very early the difference between knowing the name of something and knowing something."*

Abdullah A. Alabdulgader, MD, DCH, MRCP, FRCP

Why The International Network of Cholesterol Skeptics, THINCS, Was Created

Uffe Ravnskov, MD, PhD

Progress in science demands curiosity and questioning, but curiosity and questioning of established wisdom is not welcome in the medical world. It is very difficult to convince a professor who has believed in a hypothesis and argued for it for many years that he or she has been wrong; particularly if he or she has been paid generously by the drug industry. You have to be very stubborn to succeed.

I am Danish, but I have lived most of my life in Sweden. When I received my MD from the University of Copenhagen in 1961, a colleague of mine told me that according to American researchers, high cholesterol was the cause of coronary heart disease, because serum cholesterol of those dying from a heart attack is higher than normal.

I laughed loudly because I was still able to remember what I had learned about cholesterol, one of our most important molecules. One of the commonest mistakes in medical research is to claim that something which is strongly associated with a disease is the cause, but association is not the same as causation. It is not the fire brigade who put houses on fire, although almost all burning houses are surrounded by firemen. Neither is lung cancer caused by yellow fingers although many patients with lung cancer have yellow fingers.

I was sure that wiser researchers would be able to show that this idea was highly unlikely, but unfortunately, I was wrong. However, it took about 25 years before I started my research dealing with fat and cholesterol.

In the interim, I worked for 11 years in the Departments of Nephrology and Clinical chemistry at the University of Lund in Sweden. My PhD was about proteinuria (the presence of protein in the urine) and my main interest during the following years was glomerulonephritis (a disease claimed to be caused by destruction of the glomeruli; the kidney filters). Together with some of my

17

colleagues I discovered that many patients with glomerulonephritis, in particular those with kidney failure, had been exposed to chemicals that destroyed the cells of the kidney tubules, and that elimination of the exposure improved their kidney function.

All of my papers about proteinuria had been accepted without any problems, because I hadn't questioned anything; I had only introduced better methods to measure and interpret proteinuria; for instance, the albumin/creatinine ratio. At that time, all nephrologists "knew" that glomerulonephritis was an immunologic or infectious disease, and when I started questioning this idea, most of my papers were rejected.

In one study, I found that almost all of our patients with poststreptococcal glomerulonephritis (a type of glomerulonephritis that appears shortly after an infection with streptococci) had been exposed to organic solvents for several years or they had been exposed during the period between the streptococcal infection and the start of the glomerulonephritis. Half a year after the submission of the paper, it was rejected, because the editor considered my conclusion was ridiculous. How did I explain that Indians living in the forests of Trinidad got poststreptococcal glomerulonephritis? My paper was accepted by another journal however, and a few years later I read that many forested areas in Trinidad are criss-crossed by oil and gas extraction infrastructures. Probably some of the Indians had worked at these places.

That renal failure in glomerulonephritis is a result of infections is apparently supported by numerous experiments where this disease has been produced by injecting various types of microorganisms or their toxic products into experimental animals. But to succeed with producing renal failure in such experiments, it is necessary to solve the microorganisms in Freund's adjuvant, a chemical which is produced by mineral oil. Without using Freund's adjuvant, the glomerulonephritis healed in the course of a few days or weeks. In one of the experiments, renal failure was produced by injecting Freund's adjuvant alone. However, the authors didn't understand the importance of this finding; nor have any of their colleagues.

When I revealed that one of my co-workers had falsified his doctoral thesis, I came into a serious conflict with the professors and I therefore started a private practice. However, I continued my research into kidney disease and published several papers in major medical journals. Nevertheless, I have not succeeded with changing the general view about the cause of renal failure in glomerulonephritis and other kidney diseases. If you are interested, I have created a summary of my research about this issue on the web (www.ravnskov.nu/GN).

When the cholesterol campaign started in Sweden in the eighties, I became surprised because I had followed the literature superficially without finding any study showing that saturated fat or high cholesterol were unhealthy. Were the cholesterol researchers just as blindfolded as those who studied glomerulonephritis? I started to read the literature about this issue systematically and I soon realised that it was the greatest medical scandal in modern times.

The diet-heart idea and the cholesterol hypothesis had become popular in the early fifties. During that period, Ancel Keys, an American nutritionist, published several papers claiming that high cholesterol is the cause of cardiovascular disease and that a high intake of saturated fat raises cholesterol. One of his proofs was a diagram showing the association between the intake of saturated fat and serum cholesterol in different countries.

However, he did not include any references to these data, and it was easy for me to see that he had ignored observations from several African populations who ate at least twice as much saturated fat as other people on this planet and who had the lowest cholesterol ever measured in healthy people.

One of his other proofs was another diagram, which showed that intake of fat food was associated with coronary heart mortality in six countries. However, Yerushalmy and Hilleboe, two American researchers showed that once again, Keys had falsified his data. They published three diagrams. The first one was Keys´ original one where the dots from the six countries lay close to a straight line curve he had constructed. The second diagram showed the same after the American researchers had corrected his six figures, as they were available in a report from WHO. Their corrected diagram demonstrated that Keys had changed the WHO data to better fit the curve. The third diagram showed that Keys had excluded data from 16 countries and when all data were included, there was no longer any association between fat intake and heart disease.

The proof from the Framingham study wasn´t particularly convincing either, because there was a large overlapping of the two curves representing the cholesterol level among those who died from a heart disease during the first observation period and those who didn´t.

Furthermore, most cholesterol-lowering trials had been performed without having lowered the risk of heart mortality with statistical significance. Here is an example.

In MRFIT, one of the largest cholesterol-lowering trials, the upper three percent of the cholesterol range among more than 300,000 men were selected; a total of 12,000 men. Half of them were instructed every fourth month, during seven years, to stop smoking; to follow a diet low in cholesterol and saturated fat and high in polyunsaturated fat; high blood pressure was treated energetically, and subjects with weight problems were taught regularly how to reduce calories and get more exercise. The other half got no instructions or medicine. Seven years later no significant differences were noted; neither as regards nonfatal or fatal coronary disease, nor as regards total mortality.

Another example is the LRC trial. Here, cholesterol was measured in more than half a million men, after which the upper 0.8 per cent of the cholesterol range were selected; a total of about 4000 middle-aged men. As about half per cent of mankind has familial hypercholesterolemia, most of the participants must have belonged to that category. Half of them were treated with the cholesterol-lowering drug cholestyramine, the other half with a placebo (a sugar pill). The trial was ended after seven years and the result was not impressive. The authors claimed that the small differences were significant. However, they had lowered their own statistical demands. In a preliminary report, they had stated that they would accept nothing less than a p-value of 0.01 using the two-tailed t-test. But in the trial report they had shifted their demand from 0.01 to 0.05 using the one-tailed t-test, and the one-tailed t-test is only allowed if you know for certain that the result only can go in one direction. Nonetheless, the LRC trial became the official start of the cholesterol campaign.

Obviously, the supporters of the diet-heart idea and the cholesterol hypothesis misused statistics to keep the idea alive. But it is worse than that. By reading the relevant medical literature I realised that they used many other questionable methods.

In a paper published in 1990 by the American Heart Association and the U.S. National Heart, Lung and Blood Institute you can read the following: '*A one percent reduction in an individual's cholesterol results in an approximate two percent reduction in CHD (coronary heart disease) risk*', and here the authors referred to a 30-year follow-up study of the

Framingham population. I became curious because I had not yet found any study proving that high cholesterol was the cause of heart disease. What I found was that the authors lied because in the Framingham report you can read the opposite: *'For each 1 mg/dl drop in TC per year, there was an eleven percent increase in coronary and total mortality'.*

I decided to analyse two more reviews published by the supporters. Among the authors were several well-known authorities, for instance William B. Kannel, who was the director of the Framingham study and the head of the American Heart Association's Council of Epidemiology; John C. LaRosa, who was president and professor of medicine at the State University of New York Downstate Medical Center, and Scott M. Grundy, who was professor of internal medicine at the University of Texas Southwestern Medical School and who has chaired a number of American Heart Association committees. All of them have authored or co-authored several statin trials and all of them are or were paid by Big Pharma. At that time several studies had shown that the diet-heart idea and the cholesterol hypothesis did not satisfy the definition of science. To see how these proponents explained their discordant results, I searched the three reviews for quotations of 12 articles with such findings. Only two of the articles were quoted correctly and only in one of the reviews. About half of the contradictory articles were ignored. In the rest, statistically nonsignificant findings in favour of the cholesterol hypothesis were inflated, and unsupportive results were quoted as if they were supportive. Only one of the six randomized cholesterol-lowering trials with a negative outcome was cited and only in one of the reviews.

Several meta-analyses (reviews) of the many cholesterol-lowering trials have been published before the introduction of the statins. However, all of them have excluded most of the unsupportive trials. I therefore decided to perform a meta-analysis myself where I included all the trials, and my review was published in the *British Medical Journal* in 1992. Although the intervention in the treatment group in several of the trials also included physical exercise, weight loss, reduction of blood pressure and smoking advice, the number of non-fatal heart attacks was not reduced by more than 0.3 per cent, the number of fatal heart attacks was the same in both groups, and total mortality was highest in the treatment groups.

The reason why these results haven't made any influence in the medical world is that trials with apparent positive results are cited more often than trials with negative results. As an example, the LRC trial, which was claimed to be in support of the cholesterol hypothesis, was cited at that time in 612 medical papers during the first four years after its publication, whereas the Finnish Miettinen trial, where mortality was twice as high in the treatment group than in the control group, was cited in 15 papers only, although both trial reports had been published in the same journal.

Several critical responses to my meta-analysis were published in the *British Medical Journal*, and in the following years, I found that my critical papers were very difficult, if not impossible to get accepted by most medical journals.

I realized that to inform my colleagues and the public about what I today consider as the greatest medical scandal in modern time, it was necessary to write a book. It was published in Sweden in 1991 and in Finland and Denmark a few years later, and initiated intense debates in the Scandinavian media. I was ignorant, irresponsible, I hadn't researched about the issue myself; my arguments were tendentious and unilateral. One of my critics wrote that my arguments were so mad that he simply hadn't the strength to discuss them with me.

When my book was published in Finland, a Finnish journalist and photographer came to my home to interview me. Shortly after, Finnish television presented a program devoted to cholesterol. It took about a quarter of an hour, but they had only included two short sentences from the long interview with me. In the rest of the program, several Finnish professors presented the general view, and they burned my book at the end of the program.

Shortly afterwards, the first statin trial called 4S was published. For the first time a massive lowering of cholesterol was achieved in patients with cardiovascular disease. I participated in a meeting in Sweden where a representative from Merck, the drug company which had produced the statin-lowering drug, told doctors about its benefit. When he showed us the data, I saw that there was no exposure-response, meaning that the benefit was the same whether cholesterol had been lowered very much or only a little. I asked him to explain this contradictory finding, but he was unable to do so. Furthermore, in the trial report, the authors claimed that the benefit was achieved in both sexes, although total mortality was only lowered among the males. In fact, total mortality was a little higher among women in the treatment group, although not with statistical significance.

But 4S wasn't the real first statin trial. Three years before the publication of 4S, Merck published the results of a 48 weeks long trial named EXCEL which included only healthy people with high cholesterol. It consisted of five groups; four treated with different statin doses; one with placebo (a pill without any effect; usually a sugar pill). The authors' conclusion was that their drug was able to lower cholesterol and was well tolerated.

Obviously, the trial had started about the same time as 4S. But why did they end this trial after only 48 weeks? To start a trial including almost 8000 participants costs millions of dollars, and the aim with a clinical trial is not only to see whether the drug is tolerable and safe, but also whether it has any benefit. I sent this question to Merck and they answered that their goal was only to see whether their drug was tolerable.

There is another explanation. Both cancer and total mortality were highest in the treatment groups, although not with statistical significance, but had they continued, it might have become significant. This fact wasn't mentioned in the abstract or in any of the tables. You have to read the report carefully to find this information. Furthermore, whereas all other statin reports are freely available, you have to pay for the EXCEL report.

The following years at least 20 papers were published about the EXCEL trial, but they only mentioned how effectively the drug lowered cholesterol and how well it was tolerated. Not a word about the clinical outcome.

To spread the knowledge about fat and cholesterol I translated my book into English and for several years I tried to find an English or American publisher or agent, but in vain. As I had created a website, where I presented my view and my papers in detail, I included also parts of my book. By this way I got in contact with many interesting colleagues who were just as critical of the cholesterol campaign as I was. One of them was Sally Fallon, the head of Weston A. Price Foundation, and she was interested in publishing my book. In 2001, she also invited me and my wife to visit her in Washington, and here she organized several meetings where I and some of my colleagues discussed the cholesterol scandal.

I realised that to fight alone was a bad idea. Curiosity may kill the cat, but it is more difficult if it isn't alone. Therefore, I suggested that we created an organization of open-minded researchers with the aim to inform our colleagues and the general population about the benefit of saturated fat and high cholesterol and about the criminal ways by which the drug industry misleads the world. We have called it THINCS, The International Network of Cholesterol Skeptics. Today we have more than a hundred members, a third of whom are professors. We have different ideas about the cause of atherosclerosis and cardiovascular disease, but all of us have realized that it is neither saturated fat nor high cholesterol. Our homepage is available on the web (www.thincs.org).

And something is happening. If you for instance search Youtube with the words Cholesterol Myth, you will get access to hundreds of videos, where researchers tell the viewers about the cholesterol scandal.

Unfortunately, most health authorities in the world are still warning their population against saturated fat and high cholesterol, and most doctors routinely prescribe statins to patients who have suffered from a cardiovascular disease and to healthy people with high cholesterol, although this drug has numerous and serious side effects and its benefit is minimal, if present at all.

There is much evidence that the cholesterol campaign is the cause of the obesity and the diabetes epidemics that have spread to many countries. I also think that it is one of the causes, if not the most important cause of the crisis in the health care systems in many countries. For example, a few years after the official start of the campaign in the US, the obesity epidemic started and a few years later it was followed by the diabetes epidemic. The fact that statin treatment may cause serious side effects in more than 20 per cent of the treated individuals, and that millions of people all over the world have been prescribed such drugs, must have added even more health problems. As an example, I shall mention that when I moved from Denmark to Sweden in 1962, there were only about 8000 active physicians in Sweden, but it was easy to get in contact with a doctor and you didn't wait for more than a few days or weeks to be operated. Today, there are more than 40,000 active physicians in

Sweden, although the population only has increased from 8 to about 10 million. In spite of that, a cancer patient, for instance, has to wait several months to be surgically treated.

Three years ago, some of us published a review in the *British Medical Journal*, in which, based on the findings of 19 follow-up studies of elderly individuals, demonstrated that in most of them, those with the highest LDL-cholesterol live the longest, even longer than those on statin treatment; none of them found the opposite. Our paper was criticized by the statin proponents in more than a hundred newspapers all over the world, but none of them was able to point at a study with the opposite result. Instead three enormous reviews were published that were designed to support the cholesterol campaign.

In 2018, we published another paper that demonstrated the many criminal ways by which the cholesterol campaign has been kept alive. To summarize, the cholesterol hypothesis is unable to satisfy any of the Bradford Hill criteria for causality and the conclusions of the authors of the three reviews are based on misleading statistics, exclusion of unsuccessful trials and by ignoring numerous contradictory observations.

Among the more than 10,000 scientific papers with open access published that year, our paper was the most downloaded one, although it was published in October. You can read the paper here:

https://www.tandfonline.com/doi/pdf/10.1080/17512433.2018.1519391?needAccess=true

In that paper there are references to most of the studies mentioned above. More information and references are present in my books and on my website (www.ravnskov.nu). My first book (The Cholesterol Myths) is freely available on the web:

https://www.smashwords.com/books/view/486704

Furthermore, if you search YouTube with the words Cholesterol Myths, you will get access to hundreds of videos where scientists discuss various facets of the cholesterol scandal.

Uffe Ravnskov, MD, PhD

Part Two

What Causes Atherosclerosis and Coronary Heart Disease

The Competing Hypothesis – Blood Clots
(The Thrombogenic Hypothesis)

Malcolm Kendrick, MD

It may be surprising to know that there have been two hypotheses about CardioVascular Disease (CVD) battling away for well over a hundred and fifty years. In truth, it has been a bit of a one-sided contest. The cholesterol hypothesis has become so utterly dominant that it seems as if it has stood alone, unquestioned and unchallenged – indeed virtually unquestionable. Such is the way of the world. To the victor, go the spoils.

However, if you do decide to pull the curtain back, there has always been an alternative hypothesis hiding just out of sight. It has never caught the public imagination. In truth it has never seriously disturbed the views of the mainstream medical profession. Although, over the years, it has been championed quite vigorously, in different guises.

The main problem is that it is pretty much incompatible with the cholesterol hypothesis. I have seen attempts made to weld them together, but they are rather half-hearted, and splinter under a little pressure. Which means that you either believe one, or the other. I happen to believe in the other. I hope to convince you that the other is correct.

The alternative hypothesis

The alternative hypothesis is that blood clots, and blood clotting, are the key players in cardiovascular disease. From start, to finish. By which I mean that atherosclerotic plaques, the thickenings and narrowings in arteries, are the remnants of blood clots that have been deposited onto, then incorporated into, artery walls.

The process begins when the lining of the artery is disrupted in some way, by something. This stimulates the formation of a blood clot (thrombus) which covers over the area, rather like a scab does when you damage your skin. A new layer of arterial lining then grows over the top of the thrombus, which effectively draws it into the artery wall. In most cases, the remnant thrombus is then fully broken down and removed.

However, if there is an increased rate of damage, or more resilient and larger blood clots are formed, or the repair systems are not working so well, then repeated blood clotting, at the same spot, will lead to plaques getting bigger. Eventually, they will severely narrow the artery and constrict blood flow.

Over many years of growth, plaques can end up in a whole range of different forms. They can be tough and fibrous, known as fibroatheroma. They can develop an almost liquid core, like a boil, with a thin covering. These are the 'vulnerable' plaques. Such plaques are the dangerous ones, as they are more liable to rupture, exposing the plaque contents to the bloodstream which is a very powerful trigger for blood clotting.

One positive thing about plaques is that, after decades of enlarging, they normally pass through the vulnerable stage and begin to calcify. This can make them, and the surrounding artery stiff, almost like a concrete pipe. In this calcified form plaques are significantly less dangerous than earlier versions, such as the semi-liquid vulnerable plaque, as they are far less likely to rupture and trigger a heart attack, or stroke.

Almost everything written above is fully accepted by the mainstream medical community. For instance, plaque rupture causing a thrombus that can fully block an artery. This is pretty much unquestioned as the underlying cause of most heart attacks.

It is also widely accepted that thrombus formation, on top of an existing plaque, can lead to plaque enlargement. Here, for example, is a passage from a paper in the journal Atherosclerosis. The paper was called: *'The role of plaque rupture and thrombosis in coronary artery disease.'*

*'In addition, **plaque rupture and subsequent healing is recognized to be a major cause of further rapid plaque progression**.'*[1]

However, the idea that thrombi could have a role in starting the plaque in the first place is usually dismissed. It is considered to be LDL that infiltrates the arterial wall to initiate the plaque. After this, continued build-up of LDL causes further growth. It is only at the later stages that blood clotting may take over – or have some role to play.

It does seem a strange disease that can start as one process, and then transform itself into another, halfway through?

Can plaques really be blood clots?

In the mid nineteenth century Karl von Rokitansky was one of the very first researchers to look at plaques in detail. He was convinced that they represented the result of repeated deposition of blood clots.

'Rokitansky proposed that the disease is the result of an excessive intimal deposition of blood components (blood clots) including fibrin. He maintained that localized thickening, atheromatous changes and calcification of the arterial wall are due to the repeated deposition of blood elements and their subsequent metamorphosis and degeneration on the lining membrane of the vascular wall.'[2]

One of Rokitansky's key observations was the large amount of fibrin that can be found in plaques, all plaques. Fibrin is the long strand of protein that binds clots together.

Perhaps surprisingly, fibrin can be found within artery walls, when there is nothing else of a plaque to be seen:

'...in apparently healthy human subjects there appears to be a significant amount of fibrin deposited within arteries, and this should give pause for thought about the possible relationship between clotting and atherosclerosis.'[3]

How does fibrin end up within an otherwise normal arterial wall? The most likely answer is that it arrived as part of a thrombus, which was then gradually broken down and removed. The only part was fibrin. A very tough protein to break apart – without sufficient plasmin.

Finding fibrin in a healthy artery wall is like finding bones in the ground. All that remains of a dead body after the rest has rotted and been stripped away by the worms.

If we look beyond the apparently normal artery wall, it is clear that fibrin is also a key component of all plaques, right from the start, and through all stages of development:

*'Fibrin appears to be a multi-potential component of atherogenesis, intervening at virtually all stages of lesion development. Fibrin also provides a continuing source of fibrin degradation products (FDP), and these have mitogenic activity which will sustain smooth muscle cells (SMC) proliferation in growing plaques, and act as chemoattractants for blood leucocytes. **Accumulation of the lipid core in fibrous plaques may also be influenced by fibrin which appears to bind the lipoprotein Lp(a) with high affinity, thereby immobilizing its lipid moiety within the lesion.**'*[4]

In short, fibrin is incorporated into all plaques. Fibrin degradation products then act as a chemo-attractant for many other plaque components, such as macrophages. They also stimulate smooth muscle cells (SMCs) to divide and multiply. SMCs are a major component of all plaques.

In addition to this, fibrin also remains tightly bound to Lp(a), trapping the fats contained within the Lp(a) and providing the building blocks for the lipid core to develop. Finally, fibrin binds to RBCs and they, in turn, provide the 'free' cholesterol that is the building block for cholesterol crystals.

What of platelets, another key component of all blood clots?

*'Abundant evidence published from the 1960s and onwards supports the essential role of platelets in the initial stages of atherosclerosis, as recently reviewed. Governed by disturbed flow, **platelets adhere to the arterial wall in vivo, even in the absence of endothelial cell denudation, initiating lesion formation.**'*[5]

If plaques do represent blood clot after blood clot, all piled on top of another then, at least in theory, some plaques should be multi-layered. This has been confirmed in a review by the American Heart Association:

*'The architecture of some multi-layered fibroatheromas could also be explained by **repeated disruptions of the lesion surface, hematomas, and thrombotic deposits.**'*[6]

The idea that repeated thrombus formation can drive plaque growth, is reinforced by an article in the journal *Atherosclerosis*.

'In addition, plaque rupture and subsequent healing is recognized to be a major cause of further rapid plaque progression.'[7]

32

The concept is also supported by an article in the Journal: *Heart.*

'Subclinical episodes of plaque disruption followed by healing are a stimulus to plaque growth that occurs suddenly and is a major factor in causing chronic high-grade coronary stenosis. This mechanism would explain the phasic rather than linear progression of coronary disease observed in angiograms carried out annually in patients with chronic ischaemic heart disease.'[8]

Phasic, rather than linear, means that plaques do not gradually enlarge. Instead, they suddenly jump in size. How could this happen? Because a clot has formed on top of an already existing plaque, then it has been incorporated, causing the plaque to enlarge.

Dr Elspeth Smith, from Scotland is another researcher who believed that plaques formed as a result of repeated thrombus formation. The thrombogenic hypothesis.

'After many years of neglect, the role of thrombosis in myocardial infarction is being reassessed. It is increasingly clear that all aspects of the haemostatic system are involved: not only in the acute occlusive event, but also in all stages of atherosclerotic plaque development from the initiation of atherogenesis to the expansion and growth of large plaques.'[9]

It can be strongly argued, therefore, that plaques truly are the remnants of repeated thrombus deposition within the artery wall.

The thrombogenic process in more detail

The first step is that the endothelium is damaged in some way, by something. After this, a blood clot forms to cover the area. Once the clot has stabilised, it is gradually shaved down in size.

Endothelial progenitor cells then move in, grow, and cover over the clot, and effectively draw it into the arterial wall. At this point, macrophages arrive (or have already arrived). They clear up the remnant blood clot, and it is gone. That, anyway, is the normal healthy process.

Problems start to happen, and a plaque will start, and continue to grow, if:

- There is an increased rate of endothelial damage

- The blood clot formed is bigger, or more difficult to break-down, than normal

- The repair systems are impaired in some way.

Which means that any factor that increases the risk of CVD will do one of the three things listed above. Perhaps all three. Plaques will also develop more rapidly if several factors are working in unison.

On the positive side, if there are protective factors in operation, then CVD will be slowed. It may even be possible to reverse the process. I shall use an analogy here, which is potholes in the road.

Road surfaces are under constant attack from rain, ice, tractor tyres, car tyres, direct sunlight and suchlike. Over time they will start to break down, cracks and potholes will develop. Then the potholes will get bigger and bigger.

If the local council spends money on repair, or resurfacing, then roads will remain in good condition. If not, things can get very bad indeed. See under, UK roads, currently.

Essentially, what we have, with roads, is an on-going battle between damage and repair. If repair > damage, then all is well. If damage > repair, then things will end badly. Cyclists will disappear into huge potholes and suchlike. Car tyres will blow up – I speak from bitter experience here.

The same thing is happening in arteries. If repair > damage, then all is well. But if damage > repair then atherosclerotic plaques can develop. This is why age is the single most important risk factor for CVD. As we age, the rate of damage may not worsen. However, the repair systems start to fail in several different ways.

For example:

'Age decreases endothelial progenitor cell recruitment.'[10]

'Experimental models suggest that endothelium-derived nitric oxide is reduced with aging, and this reduction is implicated in atherogenesis.'[11]

The thrombogenic hypothesis and various risk factors

If the thrombogenic hypothesis is correct, then it should be able to explain how various risk factors can increase CVD risk.

There are very large number of these, so in this chapter I will restrict myself to looking at seven, which make up part of the algorithm used in UK Qrisk3 calculator https://qrisk.org/three/. The reason for choosing these seven is that they do not appear, at least superficially, to be in any way related to each other. They are certainly not explained by the cholesterol hypothesis.

However, they can be simply fitted together within the thrombogenic hypothesis. They are:

- Smoking

- Diabetes

- Raised blood pressure

- Chronic Kidney Disease

- Systemic Lupus Erythematosus (SLE)

- Using steroid tablets

- History of migraines.

Before exploring them in further detail I want to highlight three critical players in plaque causation, or prevention of plaques. These are nitric oxide, endothelial progenitor cells (EPCs) and the glycocalyx.

Nitric oxide has many protective effects. It stimulates EPC growth in the bone marrow, protects the endothelial cells, and it also acts as a powerful anticoagulant.

'Adequate levels of endothelial NO are important to preserve normal vascular physiology – in the face of diminished NO bioavailability, there is endothelial dysfunction, leading to increased susceptibility to atherosclerotic disease.'[12]

Endothelial progenitor cells are critical for the effective repair of damaged endothelium. They are attracted to areas of vascular damage, they then cover over the resultant damage and form a new layer of endothelium:

'Endothelial progenitor cells (EPCs) move towards injured endothelium or inflamed tissues and incorporate into foci of neovascularisation, thereby improving blood flow and tissue repair. **Patients with cardiovascular diseases have been shown to exhibit reduced EPC number and function.**'[13]

The glycocalyx is a 'forest' of glycoproteins that lines all endothelial cells and protects them from damage.

The glycocalyx:

- Forms the interface between the vessel wall and moving blood

- Acts as the exclusion zone between blood cells and the endothelium

- Acts as a barrier against leakage of fluid, proteins and lipids across the vascular wall

- Interacts dynamically with blood constituents

- Acts as the "molecular sieve" for plasma proteins

- Modulates adhesion of inflammatory cells and platelets to the endothelial surface

- Functions as a sensor and mechano-transducer of the fluid shear forces to which the endothelium is exposed; thus, the glycocalyx mediates shear-stress-dependent nitric oxide production

- Retains protective enzymes (e.g. superoxide dismutase)

- Retains anticoagulation factors, e.g.: Tissue factor inhibitor, Protein C, Nitric Oxide (NO), Antithrombin.[14]

Damage to the glycocalyx exposes the underlying endothelial cells to toxins and will accelerate endothelium damage.

Therefore, if the thrombogenic hypothesis is correct, any factor that can reduce NO synthesis, or EPC numbers, or damage the glycocalyx and/or the underlying endothelium will greatly increase the risk of CVD.

Smoking

Smoking a cigarette causes many nanoparticles to find their way into the bloodstream, where they can attack the endothelium. This damage does not take years to build up, it is virtually instantaneous.

A healthy volunteer, smoking a single cigarette, can kill enough endothelial cells for their remnants to be measured in a blood test. These endothelial cells remnants are called microparticles (MPs). A sudden increase in microparticles indicates that endothelial cells have died.

The good news for cigarette smokers is that the death of endothelial cells simultaneously triggers the production of new Endothelial Progenitor Cells (EPCs) in the bone marrow. So, the repair system kicks immediately.

For example, a study in volunteers found that:

*'Brief active smoking of one cigarette generated an **acute release of EPC and MPs** (microparticles), of which the latter contained nuclear matter. Together, these results demonstrate acute effects of cigarette smoke on **endothelial, platelet and leukocyte function as well as injury to the vascular wall.'* [15]

Another review on the impact of smoking demonstrated that:

*'Vascular dysfunction induced by smoking is initiated by **reduced nitric oxide (NO) bioavailability** and further by the increased expression of adhesion molecules and subsequent **endothelial dysfunction**. Smoking-**induced increased adherence of platelets and macrophages provokes the development of a procoagulant** and inflammatory environment.'* [16]

In short, smoking a cigarette instantly triggers at least two of the three 'thrombogenic' processes. Endothelial damage, and the stimulation of blood clots.

Other air pollutants, such as diesel exhaust fumes can have the same effect.

'There is a **proven link between exposure to traffic-derived particulate air pollution and the incidence of platelet-driven cardiovascular diseases**. It is *suggested that inhalation of small, nanosized particles increases cardiovascular risk via toxicological and inflammatory processes and* **translocation of nanoparticles into the bloodstream has been shown in experimental models...** *This study provides a potential mechanism for the* **increased thrombotic risk** *associated with exposure to ambient particulate air pollution.'* [17]

Diabetes

Diabetes/hyperglycaemia has several damaging effects:

- Reduced NO synthesis[18]

- Endothelial damage[19]

- Increased blood coagulation[20]

- A reduction in EPCs.[21]

But with diabetes, the damage does not stop here. A high blood sugar (hyperglycaemia) creates another major problem, which is that it seriously damages the glycocalyx. The low friction protective layer, covering your endothelium. This, in turn, exposes the underlying endothelium.

This effect was highlighted in the paper: '*Loss of endothelial glycocalyx during acute hyperglycemia coincides with endothelial dysfunction and coagulation activation in vivo.*'

'**Hyperglycemia is associated with increased susceptibility to atherothrombotic stimuli.** *The glycocalyx, a layer of proteoglycans covering the endothelium, is involved in the protective capacity of the vessel wall.* **We therefore evaluated whether hyperglycemia affects the glycocalyx, thereby increasing vascular vulnerability...**

'*In the present study, we showed that the glycocalyx constitutes a large intravascular compartment in healthy volunteers that can be estimated in a reproducible fashion in vivo. More importantly, we showed that* **hyperglycemic clamping elicits a profound reduction in glycocalyx volume** *that coincides with* *increased circulating plasma levels of glycocalyx constituents like hyaluronan, an observation that is consistent with the release of glycocalyx constituents into the circulation.*[22]

In short, if the blood sugar rises too high, the glycocalyx is stripped off. This also represents the underlying cause of the widespread microvascular disease (MVD) seen in diabetes. This microvascular disease then leads on to neuropathy, retinopathy and nephropathy.

Raised blood pressure

The fact that plaques never, naturally, form in veins and only develop in the pulmonary circulation when there is underlying pulmonary hypertension, is strong evidence that the blood pressure must be above a certain level for plaques to develop.

It is also known that plaques tend to develop at bifurcations. A high blood pressure, at points of bifurcation is where the biomechanical stress on the endothelium is at its greatest. Therefore, endothelial damage is more likely to occur. Which is why a raised blood pressure is a risk factors for CVD.

Chronic Kidney Disease

With Chronic Kidney Disease (CKD) a whole series of factors interact with each other. Diabetes, CVD, hypertension, and CKD itself. Which makes this area very difficult to disentangle. How can you know which one is causing the other? If one gets worse, it tends to drag the others with it.

However, it does seem to be the case that, once it has developed, CKD can go on to accelerate CVD independently. This is almost certainly because people with CKD are found to have seriously impaired NO synthesis, and reduced EPC synthesis:

'Earlier studies have reported that NO production is decreased in CKD and multiple mechanisms were found to be involved in causing NO deficiency in these patients.

Decreased production or reduced bioavailability of nitric oxide (NO) can result in endothelial dysfunction (ED).'[23]

Closely related to this, there is a loss of EPC production:

'In conclusion, patients with CKD have reduced numbers of circulating **CD34+ EPCs**, *which decrease progressively with advancing disease severity and increasing serum urea levels. EPC dysfunction results in a functional impairment in cell adherence and endothelial outgrowth formation (endothelial dysfunction)'* [24].

Systemic Lupus Erythematosus (SLE)

Systemic Lupus Erythematosus (SLE) carries a very high risk of CVD death.

'Traditional Framingham cardiovascular risk factors do not account for the entire risk in patients with SLE, with a shockingly higher risk among patients with SLE after adjusting for the following traditional risk factors: relative risk is 10.1 for nonfatal MI, 17.0 for death due to coronary heart disease (CHD), 7.5 for overall CHD, and 7.9 for stroke.'

Stripping these figures out. Here is the increased risk of cardiovascular disease in SLE:

Non-fatal MI	= 910%
Death due to CHD/MI	= 1,600%
Death from overall CVD	= 650%
Death due to stroke	= 690%[25]

If you restrict the analysis to younger women the increase in risk is far, far, greater: Increased risk of death from CVD in younger women = **4,900%**.[26]

The reason for the increased risk is almost certainly because SLE causes a severe vasculitis. Which can also be thought of as severe endothelial damage. The resultant endothelial damage leads to inflammation and significant thrombus formation:

'The relationship between inflammation and thrombosis is not a recent concept, but it has been largely investigated only in recent years. **Nowadays inflammation-induced thrombosis is considered to be a feature of systemic autoimmune diseases such as Systemic Lupus Erythematosus (SLE), Rheumatoid Arthritis (RA), or Sjögren Syndrome (SS).'** [27]

As can be seen from the quote above, vasculitis and inflammation are also a feature of other conditions such as rheumatoid arthritis and Sjögren Syndrome – which also cause an increased risk in CVD. As indeed, do all other forms of vasculitis.

The reason why SLE leads to the greatest increase in CVD death, is almost certainly because it is often associated with antiphospholipid syndrome (APS)[28]. This is a condition whereby the phospholipids in the endothelial cells membrane are attacked by the immune system, leading to significant endothelial cell damage – and blood clots forming.

Using steroid tablets

Steroids are all synthesized from the basic corticosteroid hormone, cortisol. Cortisol, in excess has a wide range of potentially damaging metabolic effects. Perhaps the most important is that cortisol/corticosteroids are direct antagonists to insulin at most sites in the body. This leads to insulin resistance, the metabolic syndrome and, often, frank type II diabetes.

Which is why Cushing's disease greatly increases the risk of CVD – up to seven hundred per cent in some studies. Patients prescribed long term steroids – that can cause Cushing's syndrome – also suffer a significant increase in CVD risk.

*'Patients prescribed systemic glucocorticoids who developed iatrogenic Cushing's syndrome had nearly a **three times greater risk of cardiovascular disease**, including coronary heart disease, heart failure, and cerebrovascular disease than patients prescribed glucocorticoids who were not known to have developed a cushingoid appearance. **This risk increased to over fourfold** in comparison with people not prescribed glucocorticoids.'*[29]

History of migraines

The causal chain between migraines and CVD is somewhat less direct. However, it seems likely that most migraines can be considered a specific type of 'short-term' vasculitis. In support of this, here is a short section from a case history on a woman with Crohn's disease, who suffered severe migraines – that were traced back to vasculitis.

'A 28-year-old woman with Crohn's disease and known migraine with aura had suffered from daily migraine attacks with recurrent focal neurological deficits for 6 weeks. Cerebral magnetic resonance imaging showed multiple acute, subacute, and chronic ischemic lesions in different vascular territories. Magnetic resonance and computed tomography angiography **demonstrated vessel changes consistent with cerebral vasculitis.'**[30]

The paper was called *'Cerebral vasculitis mimicking migraine with aura in a patient with Crohn's disease.'* It is also known that other immune diseases can overlap with vasculitis and migraine.

Which means that vasculitis can mimic migraine, or that it can cause migraine? Or perhaps some migraines are caused by vasculitis, whilst others are not, but the association of migraines and CVD is due, only, to the vasculitis induced migraines?

Here is a short list of other auto-immune conditions, that can cause vasculitis, that have also been found to cause migraines:

- SLE[31]

- APS[32]

- Sjögren's disease.[33]

Looking specifically at APS, migraines are so common in this condition that it has been suggested migraine headaches should be included within the classification of the disease. As discussed in the paper *'Antiphospholipid syndrome (APS) revisited: Would migraine headaches be included in future classification criteria?'*

Therefore, it seems that vasculitis/endothelial dysfunction, hypercoagulability, migraine and CVD are part of an interrelated spectrum. A paper in the BMJ provides further support for this idea.

'Migraine is associated with ischaemic stroke and ischaemic heart disease, particularly among women and among migraine patients with aura. Potential underlying mechanisms include **endothelial dysfunction, hypercoagulability, platelet aggregation...'**[34]

Summary

This chapter is, by its nature, a rapid run through the thrombogenic hypothesis of cardiovascular disease. The ideas presented here are not new, indeed they have been around for well over one hundred and fifty years.

For various reasons, it has been never managed to overturn the cholesterol hypothesis. However, I believe that it fits the known facts about CVD far better than the cholesterol hypothesis.

It can also explain why such diverse causal factors as: smoking, diabetes, SLE and migraine – to name only four – can increase the risk of CVD. Factors where the cholesterol hypothesis does not have any part to play.

I believe that the time has come for the mainstream thinking on CVD to move away from cholesterol, and back to the thrombogenic hypothesis.

Malcolm Kendrick, MD

General Practitioner in the UK
Independent Researcher
www.drmalcolmkendrick.org

References

1. https://www.sciencedirect.com/science/article/pii/S0021915099004797

2. Pathobiology of the Human Atherosclerotic Plaque. ISBN-14: 978-1-4612-7968-6. Seymour Glabog, Williman P Newmman III, Sheldon A. Schaffer, pp. 360.

3. https://www.sciencedirect.com/sdfe/pdf/download/eid/1-s2.0-0049384894900493 /first-page-pdf

4. https://www.ncbi.nlm.nih.gov/pubmed/8379153

5. https://onlinelibrary.wiley.com/doi/pdf/10.1111/j.1538-7836.2008.02867.x

6. https://www.ahajournals.org/doi/full/10.1161/01.CIR.92.5.1355

7. https://www.sciencedirect.com/science/article/pii/S0021915099004797

8. https://www.ncbi.nlm.nih.gov/pmc/articles/PMC1729162/

9. https://www.sciencedirect.com/sdfe/pdf/download/eid/1-s2.0-0049384894900493 /first-page-pdf

10. https://www.ahajournals.org/doi/full/10.1161/CIRCULATIONAHA.107.715847

11. https://link.springer.com/article/10.1007/BF02874163

12. https://academic.oup.com/cardiovascres/article/77/1/19/463897

13. https://new.hindawi.com/journals/bmri/2013/845037/

14. https://derangedphysiology.com/main/required-reading/infectious-diseases-antibiotics-and-sepsis/Chapter%201.3.1/significance-endothelial-glycocalyx

15. https://www.ncbi.nlm.nih.gov/pmc/articles/PMC3938677/

16. https://www.ncbi.nlm.nih.gov/pubmed/24554606

17. https://www.ncbi.nlm.nih.gov/pubmed/23206187

18. https://diabetes.diabetesjournals.org/content/62/8/2645

19. https://www.sciencedirect.com/science/article/pii/S0925443913002718

20. https://onlinelibrary.wiley.com/doi/full/10.1111/j.1538-7836.2008.03185.xetc.

21. https://www.researchgate.net/publication/225080784_Type_2_diabetes_mellitus_is_associated_with_an_imbalance_in_circulating_endothelial_and_smooth_muscle_progenitor_cell_numbers

22. https://diabetes.diabetesjournals.org/content/55/2/480

23. https://www.ncbi.nlm.nih.gov/pmc/articles/PMC4588324/

24. https://journals.physiology.org/doi/full/10.1152/ajprenal.90755.2008

25. https://www.ncbi.nlm.nih.gov/pubmed/11665973

26. https://www.frontiersin.org/articles/10.3389/fmed.2018.00200/full

27. https://www.ncbi.nlm.nih.gov/pmc/articles/PMC4399148/

28. https://www.healthline.com/health/hughes-syndrome

29. https://www.bmj.com/content/345/bmj.e4928

30. https://www.ncbi.nlm.nih.gov/pubmed/19402574

31. https://www.hopkinslupus.org/lupus-info/lupus-affects-body/lupus-nervous-system/

32. https://www.ncbi.nlm.nih.gov/pubmed/27423434

33. https://www.mdedge.com/neurology/article/114974/headache-migraine/why-eye-should-be-focus-when-treating-migraine

34. https://www.bmj.com/content/360/bmj.k96

Does Inflammation Cause Coronary Atherosclerosis?

Carlos ETB Monteiro, Paul J. Rosch, MD

Abstract

It has been proposed that inflammation, as defined by an elevated hs-CRP (high sensitivity C-reactive protein), causes coronary atherosclerosis and contributes to numerous other diseases. However, this inflammation is a response to injury to the endothelial layer of the coronary arteries, which can be due to infections and other irritants. In addition, if inflammation caused coronary heart disease, then why did powerful nonsteroidal anti-inflammatory drugs increase heart attacks in low risk patients? This inflammatory process cannot be felt or seen, in contrast to the heat, swelling, pain and redness of inflammation as it was defined by Celsus, so perhaps it should be called something else to avoid confusion. This article will discuss various influences that affect inflammation, such as the pivotal role of sympathetic nervous system stimulation and humoral influences that also regulate heart rate and other vital functions. In that regard, studies show that inflammation is associated with an increase in heart rate as well as reduced heart rate variability, a powerful predictor of risk for coronary heart disease and sudden cardiac death. Inflammation is also associated with an increased acid environment due to metabolic acidosis, which affects the function of monocytes and macrophages that modulate immune system responses. Stimulation of the sympathetic nervous system also promotes glycolysis and increases lactic acid and lactate production that further lower pH. In contrast, stimulation of the vagus nerve and parasympathetic activities have anti-inflammatory effects that provide significant benefits in patients with rheumatoid arthritis, depression and other diseases that are unresponsive to conventional therapies. We will discuss the role of canakinumab in heart disease patients with an elevated hs-CRP signifying increased inflammation, as revealed in the CANTOS trial. Canakinumab is a monoclonal antibody that lowers hs-CRP and inhibits interleukin-1β, another marker of inflammation. Although both were lowered, the treated group had more deaths from infection and the US FDA rejected the request for the treatment of heart disease. We will also discuss Omega-3 fatty acids, the surprising anti-inflammatory effects of cardiac glycosides, and the role of lactate and acidosis.

Atherosclerosis and Inflammation

There have been increasing claims that coronary atherosclerosis is due to a silent *"low-grade chronic inflammation."* This is associated with an increase in hs-CRP (high sensitivity C-reactive protein), which measures levels much lower than the traditional CRP test used for more than eight decades to assess the degree of acute inflammation. Over 2000 years ago, Celsus defined inflammation as heat, swelling, redness and pain. But all of these can be seen or felt, whereas this subtle chronic inflammation produces no signs or symptoms. Nor does it respond to anti-inflammatory drugs or antibiotics. It has also been proposed that hs-CRP actually causes inflammation and coronary atherosclerosis, rather than being a mere marker like high LDL and low HDL.

The JUPITER rosuvastatin trial contradicted this, since although LDL-cholesterol (LDL-c) was reduced by 50%, the largest drop in any statin trial, and hs-CRP was lowered by 37%, there were more fatal heart attacks in the statin treatment group. Moreover, as noted above, reducing inflammation does not reduce heart disease. Vioxx, a powerful non-steroidal anti-inflammatory drug, was taken off the market because it caused heart attacks, and other anti-inflammatory drugs have similar effects.[1]

Rudolph Virchow, who first noted the presence of cholesterol in atheroma, described what would later be called atherosclerosis as *"endarteritis deformans"*.[2] The "itis" signified inflammation, because he did not believe that atherosclerosis was due to the deposition of cholesterol, since this came later.

Van Haller used the Greek word *"atheroma"* to refer to a gruellike material in 1775, but "atherosclerosis" did not appear until 1904, when Marchand coined it to indicate a hardening of this material in the walls of arteries. A few years earlier, Lobstein had introduced arteriosclerosis to depict a calcification of these arterial lesions as they aged.

Vascular calcifications can be classified into two separate types depending on whether they are located within the intimal or medial layer. Medial arterial calcification primarily affects the legs and is prevalent in patients with peripheral vascular disease. Intimal calcification predominates in coronary vessels. While both types can be found in the carotid arteries and they share some features, they have different causes and consequences.

Although atherosclerosis and arteriosclerosis are relatively recent terms, these disorders are not new. CT analyses of Egyptian mummies and other ancient cultures where corpses were well preserved due to very dry or cold conditions, such as the Peruvian Incas, the Aleutian Island Unangans and the Ancestral Puebloans of southwest America, reveal that they were not uncommon 3500 to 4000 years ago, especially in the elderly and elite. Atherosclerosis was regarded as definite if a calcified plaque was seen in the wall of an artery, and probable if it was seen along the expected course of an artery. Most of this calcification occurs in large vessels like the aorta, iliac and carotid arteries. It is primarily medial arteriosclerosis since the deposits are found in the muscular middle layer of the arterial wall, and is often called Mönckeberg's sclerosis, after Johann Georg Mönckeberg, who first described it in 1903. Although it differs from coronary atherosclerosis, it is likely that was also prevalent in individuals who lived longer.

The Autonomic Nervous System And Inflammation

The involuntary nervous system maintains stability in the body whenever homeostasis is threatened via its complementary but antagonistic sympathetic and parasympathetic constituents. The sympathetic nervous system and its neurotransmitters are stimulated during acute stress, which results in an increase in heart rate and blood pressure and a host of other activities throughout the body to facilitate "fight or flight".

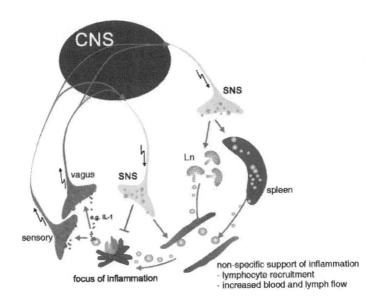

Sympathetic Nervous System Responses to Inflammation. As shown above, local inflammation is detected by vagal and sensory nerve fibers that have receptors for inflammatory mediators like interleukin and a signal sent to the brain's central nervous system (CNS) that leads to activation of the sympathetic nervous system (SNS) and the release of neurotransmitters like noradrenaline at the site, which has an anti-inflammatory effect that is a transient response to a local threat.

There is a marked increase in neutrophils, white cells that inactivate bacteria and their toxic products and promote tissue repair. Stimulation of the hypothalamic-pituitary-adrenal axis causes a rise in the secretion of cortisol that initially reduces inflammation, but this only lasts for a day or two. This contrasts with chronic systemic inflammation, which can evoke a cascade of non-specific responses such as recruitment of lymphocytes, white cells that can recognize and respond to antigens by producing antibodies. There is also increased lymph and blood flow to the affected areas. When inflammation persists and becomes chronic, the sympathetic nervous system and hypothalamic-pituitary-adrenal responses continue to be activated, but the anti-inflammatory effects of cortisol and other glucocorticoids dwindle, which ultimately results in tissue damage and organ dysfunction. Macrophages, fibroblasts, mast cells, monocytes and other immune system cells and cytokines can also contribute to this.

The parasympathetic nervous system also modulates chronic inflammation by vagal stimulation through the cholinergic anti-inflammatory pathway.

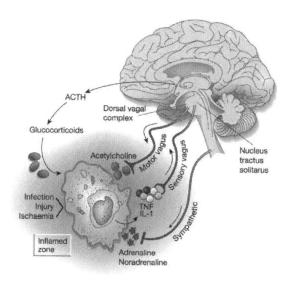

Autonomic Nervous System Responses To Inflammation. As seen to the right, inflammatory products and debris produced by damaged tissues activates afferent signals that are transmitted to the nucleus tractus solitarius. Subsequent stimulation of vagus efferent activity inhibits cytokine synthesis via the anti-inflammatory cholinergic pathway. Information can also be relayed to the hypothalamus as well as the dorsal vagal complex to stimulate the production of ACTH by the anterior pituitary. This results in an increased secretion of glucocorticoid hormones like cortisol that also decrease inflammation.

These observations have led to the development of new approaches to treating inflammation, such as modulating vagus nerve activity, or targeting specific components of this complex pathway. Meditation, biofeedback and other stress reduction measures, as well as hypnosis or acupuncture also have the potential to modulate vagal output. A variety of non-steroidal anti-inflammatory and psychoactive drugs could be designed to stimulate macrophage cholinergic receptors in the periphery or to increase vagal output comparable to a pharmacological vagus nerve stimulator. Vagal nerve stimulation has resulted in spectacular results in rheumatoid arthritis that is resistant to all other therapies and has none of their adverse side effects or addictive tendencies. It may also be effective in Crohn's disease and other inflammatory bowel disorders, as well as drug resistant depression. This non-invasive treatment is administered by the patient at home, and the dosage, frequency and duration of stimulation can easily be changed as needed.

Support for the protective effect of the parasympathetic nervous system in preventing or reducing inflammation and atherosclerosis can be found in numerous articles, and excerpts or synopses from some, are appended below:

2007 – *"Based on converging evidence, we propose a neuroimmunomodulation approach to atherogenesis. In this model, the vagus nerve 'informs' the brain about coronary artery disease related cytokines; in turn, activation of the vagus (via vagus nerve stimulation, vagomimetic drugs or relaxation) induces an anti-inflammatory response that can slow down the chronic process of atherogenesis."*[3]

2011 – *"It is also likely that in the future, the currently available treatment regimens for coronary heart disease, cardiac arrhythmias and atherosclerosis could be combined with vagus nerve stimulation and nicotinic acetylcholine receptor α7 subunit agonists."*[4]

2012 – *"The inflammatory reflex mediated by the vagus nerve has been successfully exploited therapeutically in preclinical models of diseases with aetiologies characterized by excessive inflammatory responses"*, and that *"Insufficient efferent vagus nerve cholinergic output might have a causative role in the dysfunctional immune and metabolic regulation observed in obesity, as selective activation of the efferent cholinergic arm of the inflammatory reflex attenuates both inflammation and metabolic derangements."*[5]

2014 – *"Central cholinergic activation of a vagus nerve-to-spleen circuit controls alleviates intestinal inflammation."*[6]

2016 – Vagus nerve stimulation inhibits cytokine production and attenuates disease severity in rheumatoid arthritis.[7]

Regulation of Inflammation by the Sympathetic Nervous System and Acidosis

2012 – *"Extracellular acidosis downregulates most of the hemostatic platelet functions and promotes those involved in amplifying the neutrophil-mediated inflammatory response."* (Platelet aggregation at sites of vascular injury is considered essential for hemostasis and arterial thrombosis.)[8]

2012 – *"The discovery that cholinergic neurons inhibit acute inflammation has qualitatively expanded our understanding of how the nervous system modulates immune responses. The nervous system reflexively regulates the inflammatory response in real time, just as it controls heart rate and other vital functions."*[9]

2013 – Data are provided suggesting that an acidic environment represents a novel endogenous danger signal alerting the innate immunity. *"Low pH may thus contribute to inflammation in acidosis-associated pathologies, such as atherosclerosis and post-ischemic inflammatory responses."*[10]

2014 – *"Over the past decades evidence has accumulated clearly demonstrating a pivotal role for the sympathetic nervous system (SNS) and its neurotransmitters in regulating inflammation."* The authors concluded *"However, if a 'chronic inflammatory configuration' persists, as in autoimmunity, the effects are detrimental because of the persistently increased SNS activity, HPA activity, and the resultant chronic catabolic state. This leads to known comorbidities in chronic inflammatory disease, like cachexia, high blood pressure, insulin resistance, and increased cardiovascular mortality. The challenge is now to translate this conceptual knowledge into clinical benefit."*[11]

2016 – Study demonstrating that moderate extracellular acidosis, which is a common finding in different pathological conditions such as inflammation, ischemia or in solid growing tumors, affects the functional behavior of monocytes and macrophages, and can therefore modulate the immune response.[12]

Canakinumab Anti-inflammatory Therapy and Atherosclerosis

One of the highlights of the August 2017 European Society of Cardiology Congress was the landmark CANTOS (Canakinumab Anti-inflammatory Thrombosis Outcome Study) showing that decreasing inflammation, even in the absence of any lipid lowering, significantly reduced recurrent cardiovascular events in patients with a history of myocardial infarction and an hs-CRP of two mg or more per liter. It also reduced cancer incidence and mortality.[13] Canakinumab is currently indicated for the treatment of interleukin-1ß associated inflammatory diseases, and this study allegedly provided strong support for the belief that inflammation caused recurrent coronary events because it increased atherosclerosis. In fact, the title of the paper that was published in the September 21, 2017 *New England Journal of Medicine* was "Anti-inflammatory Therapy with Canakinumab for Atherosclerotic Disease."[14]

However, the reduction in recurrent cardiovascular event rates showed only a 2% absolute risk reduction study over median follow-up of 3.7 years, Canakinumab was associated with a higher incidence of fatal infections compared to placebo and there was no significant difference in all-cause mortality. In addition, the $16,000-per-dose price tag meant that treatment would cost approximately $200,000 per year, and many doctors also expressed concerns about the future of this drug based on the study results. Some argued that the same results might have been obtained with existing and much less expensive drugs.[15] In October 2018 the FDA declined to approve Canakinumab for cardiovascular risk reduction based on the CANTOS results.[16]

Not mentioned was the fact that numerous studies have shown that C-Reactive Protein is elevated with chronic stress as well as inflammation. Danish researchers also found that higher hs-CRP blood levels were associated with a greater risk of psychological stress and especially clinical depression. As the lead author noted, "*Irrespective of other factors, we found that basically healthy people with hs-CRP levels above three milligrams per liter had a two- to threefold increased risk of depression. Dampening inflammation may be one way of treating depression.*" It is not clear what explains this association, but the authors suggest that elevated CRP levels may indicate elevated levels of certain cytokines that can increase feelings of stress, or that depression itself may lead to increased inflammation.[17]

Myocardial ischemia provoked in the laboratory during acute mental stress in patients with stable coronary artery disease predicts subsequent clinical events, much like exercise induced ischemia with treadmill stress tests, but the mechanisms responsible for this are different. While sympathetic nervous system activation may play a role, little is known about how mental stress increases risk for coronary events. Since an elevated hs-CRP is also a risk marker for future coronary events in patients with heart disease, perhaps increased inflammation was responsible. To evaluate this, 83 patients with stable heart disease underwent simultaneous single-photon emission computed tomography (SPECT) and transthoracic echocardiography (TTE) at rest, and during laboratory induced mental stress. Serum hs-CRP levels were measured before and 24 hours after mental stress. Of the 83 patients, 30 (36%) showed ischemic changes due to mental stress. There was no difference in gender, sex, BMI, histories of diabetes, hypertension, smoking, lipid profile, medications used (including statins, β-blockers, ACE inhibitors, and aspirin), or hemodynamic responses during mental stress between this group and those who had no evidence of ischemia. However, they did show a greater increase in hs-CRP, and each 1 mg/L increase in this level was associated with a 20% higher risk of mental stress induced ischemia.[18] However, this does not prove that either hs-CRP or inflammation cause heart disease, since association never proves causation. Other studies have found that emotional stress can provoke ischemia in 30%–50% of patients with chronic, stable coronary disease.[19, 20]

Chronic stress, especially job stress,[21] socioeconomic status,[22] as well as social and personality factors have also been associated with increased risk of coronary heart disease as well as atherosclerotic progression.[23] Acute stress, whether provoked by national emergencies[24, 25] or severe anger[26-29] have been associated with triggering cardiac events and heart failure.[30] While mental stress–induced ischemic episodes are good indicators of 5-year rates of cardiac events,[31] stress-induced ischemia without angina occurs much more frequently than appreciated.[32-33] There is also evidence that acute stress events such as public speaking and anger-provoking situations can disrupt cardiac electrical signalling and lead to arrhythmias and other acute cardiac events, including myocardial infarction.[34]

Cardiac Glycosides, Omega-3 Fatty Acids and Acidosis

The anti-inflammatory and beneficial effects of digoxin and other cardiac glycosides have been known for decades.[35-42] A 2009 study concluded "Digitoxin elicits anti-inflammatory and vasoprotective properties. These observations indicate a potential therapeutic application of digitoxin in the treatment of cardiovascular diseases, such as atherosclerosis."[36] Another review that discussed this and other cardiac glycosides and their mechanisms of action by providing *"an overview of the in vivo and in vitro actions of cardiac glycosides on inflammatory processes and of the signalling mechanisms responsible for these effects: cardiac glycosides have been found to decrease inflammatory responses in different animal models of acute and chronic inflammation. Regarding the underlying mechanisms most research has focused on leukocytes. In these cells, cardiac glycosides primarily inhibit cell proliferation and the secretion of proinflammatory cytokines"*.[35] It is not generally appreciated that glycosides like digoxin,[43] digitoxin,[44] and ouabain[45] inhibit the sympathetic nervous system when administered in low dosages. A study done over 50 years ago showed that they inhibited epinephrine induced glycolysis and glycogenesis in skeletal muscle.[46] A more recent one demonstrated that they also inhibited lactate production and glycolysis in lung cancer cells, which require glucose, and increase the cytotoxicity of platinum compounds that are frequently used to treat lung cancer.[47] Other drugs or factors might provide similar benefits. Omega-3 fatty acids inhibit atherosclerosis without lowering cholesterol or triglycerides,[48] and some, like docosahexaenoic acid, can improve heart rate variability and baroreflex sensitivity via effects on the autonomic nervous system.[49] However, their ability to lower elevated blood lactic acid levels,[50, 51] may be even more important with respect to inhibiting coronary atherosclerosis.

Lactic Acidosis, Inflammation and Coronary Atherosclerosis

It has been known since 1934 that *"Acidity of the environment is increased in inflammatory sites."*[52] Over a half century ago, it was proposed that osteoporosis was due to an "acid ash" die, and that this was

54

buffered by bone minerals.[53] A review of this issue in 2018 confirmed that even subtle chronic acidosis can cause appreciable bone loss if prolonged.[54] In another chapter in this book, it was demonstrated that lactic acidosis is associated with coronary disease and atherosclerosis, and explained why it increases coronary artery calcification. This is consistent with the acidity theory of atherosclerosis[55, 56] that also explains how stress can cause coronary atherosclerosis.[57] It proposes autonomic dysfunction as a precursor, and particularly stimulation of the sympathetic nervous system. This increases the secretion of adrenaline and noradrenaline, which accelerates glycolysis, and results in higher concentrations of lactic acid and lactate in blood, other body fluids and tissues. Conversely, stimulation of the parasympathetic system has anti-inflammatory effects. Other factors such as age, genes, gender, lifestyle and various drugs can also influence the positive or negative effects of autonomic activities.

Association never proves causation, and as others have warned, *"Correlation implies association, but not causation. Conversely, causation implies association, but not correlation."*[58] Association should not be confused with causality unless it is clear that A always causes B and there is no other cause. Tuberculosis is one example, since it can only be caused by the tubercle bacillus, so this is not a theory but a fact. However, A and B could also be associated but not interdependent, because they are both caused by something else. An elevated cholesterol and hypertension are associated with coronary atherosclerosis, but are not always present, since this is a multifaceted disorder that can have many associated risk markers. Unlike tuberculosis, there is no vera causa or solitary true cause so that all other explanations are merely theories.

As the famous philosopher Karl Popper stated, *"A medical hypothesis cannot be proved, but it can be falsified. If it cannot be falsified, it is not a scientific hypothesis."*[59] The prevailing hypothesis that cholesterol causes coronary atherosclerosis has been refuted so many times, that it is no longer tenable. It has been replaced by a process that has been labelled inflammation, but bears no resemblance to its definition by Celsus, since it has no signs or symptoms. It can only be detected by elevations of hs-CRP, certain interleukins or other risk markers for inflammation, although these are not always consistent or correlative. This is hardly a new concept, since, as previously indicated, the renowned pathologist Rudolph Virchow, who first demonstrated the presence of cholesterol in atheroma, described atherosclerosis as *"endarteritis chronica deformans sive nodosa"* (chronic arterial inflammation with a deforming or knotty appearance), since this is what he saw under the microscope. The suffix "itis" signified that it resembled or was reminiscent of inflammation, but he was very careful to avoid calling it inflammation, since it had none of the *"tumor, rubor, calor"* or *"dolor"* (swelling, redness, heat, pain) components that Celsus listed, to which Virchow added *"functio laesa"* (loss of function.) What Virchow wrote was:

"We cannot help regarding the process as one which has arisen out of irritation of the parts stimulating them to new, formative actions; so far therefore it comes under our ideas of inflammation, or at least of those processes which are extremely nearly allied to inflammation.... We can distinguish a stage of irritation preceding the fatty metamorphosis, comparable to the stage of swelling, cloudiness, and enlargement which we see in other inflamed parts."[2]

In other words, inflammation was a response to injury of the "inner arterial coat" (endothelial layer) by some irritant, and the "so-called atheromatous degeneration" (cholesterol deposits) came later. Calling this asymptomatic prophlogistic disorder inflammation is confusing, and hopefully, future advances will lead to a more meaningful definition. As the Nobel Laureate Richard Feynman said, "I learned a long time ago the difference between knowing something and the name of something."

Virchow is still cited to support claims that inflammation rather than cholesterol causes atherosclerosis. Karl von Rokitansky, an eminent contemporary Austrian pathologist who also described inflammatory cells in atheroma, rejected inflammation as the cause of atherosclerosis, and proposed a thrombogenic origin due to the deposition of fibrinogen and other debris from repeated clot formation.[60]

It is interesting to notice that Hans Selye, in 1958, has shown experimentally how stress, combined with some agents, may induce myocardial necrosis where the coronary arteries are perfectly normal. He also said in his paper: *"It is noteworthy, however, that, under these circumstances, not only cardiac infarction but organic obstruction of the coronary vessels can regularly be produced by humoral means."[61]*

There are several hundred risk factors for coronary heart disease and atherosclerosis, but the vast majority are simply risk markers that show some statistical association but have no causal relationship.

Coronary heart disease is a multifactorial disorder that can have many causes, some of which, like stress, homocysteine, infections, and free radical damage may be interrelated. Numerous contributing factors that influence susceptibility range from family history, age, genetics, gender, diabetes, hypertension and smoking, to sex hormones, obesity, physical activity, and alcohol consumption. It would be inane to believe that levels of CRP, interleukins or other inflammation markers can provide an accurate assessment of all the varied negative and positive activities of these diverse agencies.

It would be equally foolish to assume that lowering CRP will safely and effectively reduce coronary mortality in healthy people. Treating an elevated CRP would simply repeat the same mistake that is still being made with LDL. As Albert Einstein warned, *"Not everything that counts can be counted, and not everything that can be counted counts."* The first part of this statement applies to CRP and LDL, which are easy to measure, but have no causal relationships. Association never proves causation. The second part pertains to our inability to define, much less measure, something that we call "inflammation", but may include several different processes that have yet to be elucidated.

We have tried to explain how acidosis, and especially lactate and lactic acidosis can contribute to inflammation and atherosclerosis. We also agree with Virchow's contention that a process resembling inflammation represents a response to endothelial irritation or injury. In addition, the latter is not due to lipid deposits, since these occurred subsequent to the *"swelling and cloudiness"* Virchow had observed.

Carlos ETB Monteiro, Paul J. Rosch, MD***

* Independent Researcher and Scientist
President, Infarct Combat Project (www.infarctcombat.org)
Fellow, The American Institute of Stress (www.stress.org)

** Clinical Professor of Medicine and Psychiatry
New York Medical College
Chairman, The American Institute of Stress (www.stress.org)

References

1. Rosch PJ, Ravnskov U. Why The Lipid Hypothesis of Coronary Heart Disease is Fallacious And Dangerous, pp. 113-136 in PJ Rosch ed. "Fat and Cholesterol Don't Cause Heart Attacks And Statins Are not the Solution". 2016; Columbus Publishing Ltd, U.K. at https://www.amazon.com/Cholesterol-Cause-Attacks-Statins-Solution/dp/190779753X

2. Virchow R. "Cellular Pathology": as based upon Physiological and Pathological Histology: Twenty lectures delivered in the Pathology Institute of Berlin, 1856. Published in 1858 at https://www.biodiversitylibrary.org/item/194064#page/64/mode/1up

3. Gidron Y, Kupper N, Kwaijtaal M, *et al.*, Vagus-brain communication in atherosclerosis-related inflammation: a neuroimmunomodulation perspective of CAD. Atherosclerosis. 2007 Dec;195(2):e1-9 at https://www.ncbi.nlm.nih.gov/pubmed/17101139

4. Undurti N Das. Vagal nerve stimulation in prevention and management of coronary heart disease. World J Cardiol. 2011 Apr 26; 3(4): 105–110 at https://www.ncbi.nlm.nih.gov/pmc/articles/PMC3082733/

5. Valentin A. Pavlov and Kevin J. Tracey. The vagus nerve and the inflammatory reflex—linking immunity and metabolism. Nat Rev Endocrinol. 2012 Dec; 8(12): 743–754 at https://www.ncbi.nlm.nih.gov/pmc/articles/PMC4082307/

6. Hong Ji, Mohammad F Rabbi, Benoit Labis *et al.* Central cholinergic activation of a vagus nerve - to spleen circuit alleviates experimental colitis. Mucosal Immunol. 2014 Mar; 7(2): 335–347 at https://www.ncbi.nlm.nih.gov/pmc/articles/PMC3859808/

7. Koopman FA, Sangeeta S, Miljko S *et al.* Vagus nerve stimulation inhibits cytokine production and attenuates disease severity in rheumatoid arthritis. PNAS, 2016: vol. 113; no. 29 at http://www.pnas.org/content/113/29/8284.long

8. Etulain J, Negrotto S, Carestia A *et al.* Acidosis downregulates platelet haemostatic functions and promotes neutrophil proinflammatory responses mediated by platelets. Thromb Haemost. 2012 Jan;107(1):99-110 at https://www.ncbi.nlm.nih.gov/pubmed/22159527

9. Tracey, K. J. The inflammatory reflex. Nature, 2012; 420(6917): 853–859 at https://www.nature.com/articles/nature01321

10. Rajamäki K, Nordström T, Nurmi K *et al.* Extracellular acidosis is a novel danger signal alerting innate immunity via the NLRP3 inflammasome. Journal of Biological Chemistry, Manuscript M112.426254, March 25, 2013 at https://www.ncbi.nlm.nih.gov/pmc/articles/PMC3650379/

11. Pongratz G and Straub RH The Sympathetic Nervous Response in Inflammation. Arthritis Res Ther.16(504) 2014 at http://www.ncbi.nlm.nih.gov/pmc/articles/PMC4396833/

12. Riemann A, Wußling H, Loppnow H *et al.* Acidosis differently modulates the inflammatory program in monocytes and macrophages. Biochimica et Biophysica

Acta (BBA) - Molecular Basis of Disease, 2016 V1862, Issue 1, pp. 72-81 at https://www.sciencedirect.com/science/article/pii/S0925443915003178?via%3Dihub

13. European Society of Cardiology Congress. CANTOS results show anti-inflammatory therapy lowers future cardiovascular events, reduces cancer incidence and mortality. 28 Aug 2017.

14. Ridker PM, Everett BM, Thuren T *et al*. Anti-inflammatory Therapy with Canakinumab for Atherosclerotic Disease. N Engl J Med 2017; 377:1119-1131 at https://www.nejm.org/doi/full/10.1056/NEJMoa1707914#t=article

15. Husten L. CardioBrief. Experts Caution on CANTOS and Canakinumab's Future. MedPage Today, August 27, 2017 https://www.medpagetoday.com/cardiology/cardiobrief/67534

16. Nicole Lou. FDA Rejects Canakinumab in CVD Prevention CANTOS data not enough to expand indication. MedPageToday. October 19, 2018 at https://www.medpagetoday.com/cardiology/prevention/75811

17. Wium-Andersen MK, Ørsted DD, Nielsen SF. *et al*. Elevated C-Reactive Protein Levels, Psychological Distress, and Depression in 73,131 Individuals. JAMA Psychiatry. 2013;70(2):176-184 at https://jamanetwork.com/journals/jamapsychiatry/fullarticle/1485898

18. Shah R, Burg MM, Vashist A et al. C-Reactive Protein and Vulnerability to Mental Stress-Induced Myocardial Ischemia. Mol Med. 2006; Nov-Dec; 12(11-12): 269–274 at https://www.ncbi.nlm.nih.gov/pmc/articles/PMC1829194/

19. Burg MM, Jain D, Soufer R, Kerns RD, Zaret BL. Role of behavioral and psychological factors in mental stress-induced silent left ventricular dysfunction in coronary artery disease. J Am Coll Cardiol. 1993;22:440–8 at https://www.ncbi.nlm.nih.gov/pubmed/8335813

20. Rozanski A, Bairey CN, Krantz DS, *et al*. Mental stress and the induction of silent myocardial ischemia in patients with coronary artery disease. N Engl J Med. 1988;318:1005–12 at https://www.ncbi.nlm.nih.gov/pubmed/3352695

21. Everson SA, Lynch JW, Chesney MA, *et al*. Interaction of workplace demands and cardiovascular reactivity in progression of carotid atherosclerosis: population based study. BMJ. 1997;314:553–8 at https://www.ncbi.nlm.nih.gov/pmc/articles/PMC2126071/

22. Hemingway H, Shipley M, Macfarlane P, Marmot M. Impact of socioeconomic status on coronary mortality in people with symptoms, electrocardiographic abnormalities, both or neither: the original Whitehall study 25 year follow up. J Epidemiol Comm Health. 2000;54:510–6 at https://www.ncbi.nlm.nih.gov/pmc/articles/PMC1731713/

23. Whiteman MC, Deary IJ, Fowkes FG. Personality and social predictors of atherosclerotic progression: Edinburgh Artery Study. Psychosom Med. 2000;62:703-14 at https://www.ncbi.nlm.nih.gov/pubmed/11020101

24. Leor J, Poole WK, Kloner RA. Sudden cardiac death triggered by an earthquake. N Engl J Med. 1996;334:413–9 at https://www.ncbi.nlm.nih.gov/pubmed/8552142

25. Meisel SR, Kutz I, Dayan KI, *et al.* Effect of Iraqi missile war on incidence of acute myocardial infarction and sudden death in Israeli civilians. *Lancet.* 1991;338:660–1 at https://www.ncbi.nlm.nih.gov/pubmed/1679475

26. Krantz DS, Sheps DS, Carney RM, Natelson BH. Effects of mental stress in patients with coronary artery disease: evidence and clinical implications. JAMA. 2000;283:1800–2 at https://jamanetwork.com/journals/jama/article-abstract/192564

27. Mittleman MA, Maclure M, Sherwood JB, *et al.* Triggering of acute myocardial infarction onset by episodes of anger. Determinants of Myocardial Infarction Onset Study Investigators . Circulation. 1995;92:1720–5 at https://www.ahajournals.org/doi/10.1161/01.CIR.92.7.1720

28. Servoss SJ, Januzzi JL, Muller JE. Triggers of acute coronary syndromes. Prog Cardiovas Dis. 2002;44:369–80 at https://www.ncbi.nlm.nih.gov/pubmed/12024335

29. Williams JE, Nieto FJ, Sanford CP, Tyroler HA. Effects of an angry temperament on coronary heart disease risk: The Atherosclerosis Risk in Communities Study. Am J Epidemiol. 2001;154:230–5 at https://www.ncbi.nlm.nih.gov/pubmed/11479187

30. Wittstein IS, Thiemann DR, Lima JAC, *et al.* Neurohumoral features of myocardial stunning due to sudden emotional stress [see comment] N Engl J Med. 2005;352:539–48 at https://www.nejm.org/doi/full/10.1056/nejmoa043046

31. Jiang, W, Babyak M, Krantz DS. *et al.* Mental stress-induced myocardial ischemia and cardiac events. Journal of the American Medical Association,1996; 275:1651–1656 at https://www.ncbi.nlm.nih.gov/pubmed/8637138

32. Modena M, Corghi F, Fantini G *et al.* Echocardiographic monitoring of mental stress test in ischemic heart disease. Clinical Cardiology 1989; 12, 21–24 at https://www.ncbi.nlm.nih.gov/pubmed/2912604

33. Deanfield J, Shea M. Kensett M. *et al.* Silent myocardial infarction due to mental stress. *Lancet* 1984; 11, 1001-1004 at https://www.ncbi.nlm.nih.gov/pubmed/6149394

34. Steptoe A and Brydon L Emotional triggering of cardiac events. Neuroscience and Biobehavioral Reviews, 2009; 33, 63–70 at https://www.ncbi.nlm.nih.gov/pubmed/18534677

35. Fürst R, Zündorf I, Dingermann T. New Knowledge About Old Drugs: The Anti-Inflammatory Properties of Cardiac Glycosides. Planta Med 2017 Aug;83(12-13):977-984 at https://www.ncbi.nlm.nih.gov/pubmed/28297727

36. Jagielska J, Salguero G, Schieffer B *et al.* Digitoxin elicits anti-inflammatory and vasoprotective properties in endothelial cells: Therapeutic implications for the treatment of atherosclerosis?, Atherosclerosis, 2009;206(2):390-6, 2009 at https://www.ncbi.nlm.nih.gov/pubmed/19446813

37. Kolkhof P, Geerts A, Schäfer S *et al.* Cardiac glycosides potently inhibits C-reactive protein synthesis in human hepatocytes. Biochem Biophys Res Commun 2010, 26;394 (1): 233-9 at https://www.ncbi.nlm.nih.gov/pubmed/20206126

38. Ihenetu K, Espinosa R, de Leon R *et al.* Digoxin and digoxin-like immunoreactive factors (DLIF) modulate the release of proinflammatory cytokines. Inflamm Res. 2008; 57(11): 519-23 at https://www.ncbi.nlm.nih.gov/pubmed/19109744

39. Shah VO, Ferguson J, Hunsaker LA, Deck LM, Vander Jagt DL. Cardiac Glycosides Inhibit LPS-induced Activation of Proinflammatory Cytokines in Whole Blood through an NF-κB-dependent Mechanism. International Journal of Applied Research in Natural Products, 2011 Vol. 4 (1), pp. 11-19 at http://citeseerx.ist.psu.edu/viewdoc/download?doi=10.1.1.1009.6603&rep=rep1&type=pdf

40. Yang Q, Huang W, Jozwik C, Lin Y, Glasman M *et al.* Cardiac glycosides inhibit TNF-alpha/NF-kappaB signaling by blocking recruitment of TNF receptor-associated death domain to the TNF receptor. Proc Natl Acad Sci USA. 5;102(27):9631-6, 2005 at http://www.pnas.org/cgi/content/full/102/27/9631

41. Tani S, Takano R, Oishi S *et al.* Digoxin Attenuates Murine Experimental Colitis by Downregulating Th17-related Cytokines. Inflamm Bowel Dis. 2017, 23(5):728-738 at https://www.ncbi.nlm.nih.gov/pubmed/28426455

42. Lee J, Baek S, Lee J *et al.* Digoxin ameliorates autoimmune arthritis via suppression of Th17 differentiation. International Immunopharmacol, 2015 V 26, Issue 1, 103–111 at https://www.ncbi.nlm.nih.gov/pubmed/25819229

43. Gheorghiade M and Ferguson D. Digoxin, a neurohormonal modulator for heart failure? Circulation, 1991; V84:N5 at https://www.ahajournals.org/doi/10.1161/01.CIR.84.5.2181

44. Fardin NM, Antonio EL, Montemor JA *et al.* Digitoxin improves cardiovascular autonomic control in rats with heart failure. Can J. Pharmacol, 2016; 94: 18 at https://www.ncbi.nlm.nih.gov/m/pubmed/27082032/

45. Gutman Y and Boonyaviroj P. Mechanism of inhibition of catecholamine release from adrenal medulla by diphenylhydantoin and by low concentration of ouabain (10 (-10) M). Arch Pharmacol 1977,296(3);293-6:at https://link.springer.com/article/10.1007/BF00498696

46. Kypson J Triner L, Nahas GG. The effects of cardiac glycosides and their interaction with catecholamines on glycolysis and glycogenolysis in skeletal muscle J Pharmacol Exp Ther, 1968;164(1): 22-30:1968 at http://jpet.aspetjournals.org/content/164/1/22.long

47. Calderón-Montaño J, Burgos-Morón E, Lopez-Lazaro M. The Cardiac Glycosides Digitoxin, Digoxin and Ouabain Induce a Potent Inhibition of Glycolysis in Lung Cancer Cells. WebmedCentral CANCER 2013;4(7);WMC004323: 2013 at https://www.webmedcentral.com/wmcpdf/Article_WMC004323.pdf

48. Back M and Hansson GK. Omega-3 fatty acids, cardiovascular risk, and the resolution of inflammation FASEB J. 2019; 33: 1536–1539 at https://www.fasebj.org/doi/10.1096/fj.201802445R

49. Abuissa H, O'Keefe JH, Harris H *et al.* Autonomic Function, Omega-3, and Cardiovascular Risk. Chest Journal, 2005; Volume 127: Issue 4 at https://journal.chestnet.org/article/S0012-3692(15)34447-0/fulltext

50. Ogilve GK, Fettman MJ, Mallinckrodt CH *et al*. Effect of fish oil, arginine, and doxorubicin chemotherapy on remission and survival time for dogs with lymphoma: A double-blind, randomized placebo-controlled study, Cancer, 2000; 88: 1016-28 at https://www.ncbi.nlm.nih.gov/pubmed/10760770

51. Manzi L, Costantini L, Molinari L *et al*. Effect of Dietary w-3 Polyunsaturated Fatty Acid DHA on Glycolytic Enzymes and Warburg Phenotypes in Cancer, BioMed Research International. 2015; 7 pages Article ID 137097 at https://www.hindawi.com/journals/bmri/2015/137097/

52. Menkin V. Studies on inflammation X. The cytolological picture of an inflammatory exudate in relation to its hydrogen's ion concentration, Am J Pathol. 1934 Mar; 10(2): 193–210 at https://www.ncbi.nlm.nih.gov/pmc/articles/PMC2062856/

53. Wachman A, Bernstein DS. Diet and osteoporosis. *Lancet*. 1968;1:958–9 at https://www.sciencedirect.com/science/article/pii/S0140673668909082

54. Frassetto L, Banerjee T, Powe N *et al*. Acid Balance, Dietary Acid Load, and Bone Effects—A Controversial Subject. Nutrients 2018, 10, 517 at https://www.ncbi.nlm.nih.gov/pmc/articles/PMC5946302/

55. Monteiro CETB. Acidic environment evoked by chronic stress: A novel mechanism to explain atherogenesis. Available from Infarct Combat Project, January 28, 2008 at http://www.infarctcombat.org/AcidityTheory.pdf

56. Monteiro CETB. Acidity Theory of Atherosclerosis – History, Pathophysiology, Therapeutics and Risk Factors – A Mini Review. Positive Health Online, Edition 226, November 2015 at http://goo.gl/AejGAV

57. Monteiro CETB. Stress as Cause of Atherosclerosis – The Acidity Theory. pp.204-225 in PJ Rosch ed. "Fat and Cholesterol Don't Cause Heart Attacks and Statins Are Not The Solution", Published by Columbus Publishing Ltd, 2016 at https://www.amazon.com/Cholesterol-Cause-Attacks-Statins-Solution/dp/190779753X

58. Altman N and Krzywinski M. Association, correlation and causation. Nature Methods, 2015; 12 : 899–900 at https://www.nature.com/articles/nmeth.3587

59. Popper K. Conjectures and Refutations: The Growth of Scientific Knowledge 1963; pp. 33-39, London, Routledge at https://science.sciencemag.org/content/140/3567/643.1

60. Rokitansky K: The Organs of Circulation: A Manual of Pathological Anatomy. Vol IV. 1855; Philadelphia, Blanchard & Lea at https://archive.org/details/manualofpatholog34rokirich

61. Selye H. The Humoral Production of Cardiac Infarcts, *British Medical Journal*, March 15: 1958. Full free text at http://www.ncbi.nlm.nih.gov/pmc/articles/PMC2028103/pdf/brmedj03094-0021.pdf

Lactic Acidosis as a Causal Factor for Arterial Calcification

Carlos ETB Monteiro

Life is a struggle, not against sin, not against the Money Power, not against malicious animal magnetism, but against hydrogen ions.

Mencken H. L., 1919

In 2005, I learned from a 1982 paper by David S. Schade about a discovery made by Carl F. Cori in 1925 that demonstrated the influence of adrenaline on lactic acid production. In his paper, Schade supported and expanded on this by supplying the following evidence that catecholamines participate in the development and/or maintenance of lactic acidosis:

1. The common association of stress and lactic acidosis;

2. The rise in plasma lactate concentration during adrenaline infusion;

3. The precipitation of lactic acidosis by adrenaline intoxication and pheochromocytoma;

4. The vasoconstrictor effects of catecholamines leading to tissue anoxia and lactic acid production.

For some reason, these findings have not attracted much attention until recently, but I found them stimulating. As a result, I began to investigate the importance of stress and resultant lactic acidosis as a possible causal role for disease. This led to various studies involving coronary artery disease, ischemic heart disease, acute myocardial infarction, cancer, stroke and rheumatoid arthritis.

The first disease I studied was coronary artery disease which, inspired by Dr Paul J. Rosch, resulted in the link between acidity and atherosclerosis in 2006 and published in 2008, with updated information about the acidity theory of atherosclerosis that was published in 2015.

Some basic information follows that may offer a better understanding about why chronic elevated catecholamine release, triggered by the autonomic nervous dysfunction, may accelerate the myocardial glycolysis leading to significant increase in lactate production:

1. Dysautonomia or autonomic dysfunction is a condition in which the autonomic nervous system does not work properly.

2. Autonomic neuropathies are a collection of syndromes and diseases affecting the autonomic neurons, either parasympathetic or sympathetic, or both.

3. The vagus nerve is the main component of the parasympathetic nervous system.

4. There are many risk factors leading to dysregulation of the autonomic nervous system, which are related with sympathetic dominance, through sympathetic over-activity or withdrawal of the parasympathetic system. Among these risk factors are stress, smoking, age, high carbohydrate diets, familial dysautonomia, etc.

5. Lactic acidosis results from increased production of lactate, the final product in the pathway of glucose metabolism. Lactate and lactic acid are not synonymous. Lactic acid is a strong acid which, at physiological pH, is almost completely ionized to lactate. The measurement of lactate concentration can also be made in cerebrospinal fluid, synovial fluid and other fluids and tissues of the body.

6. Lactate dehydrogenase (LDH) is a cytosolic enzyme involved in reversible transformation of pyruvate to lactate. It participates in anaerobic glycolysis of skeletal muscle and red blood cells, in liver gluconeogenesis and in aerobic metabolism of heart

muscle. The determination of its activity helps in the diagnosis of various diseases, because it is increased in the serum of patients suffering from myocardial infarction, acute hepatitis, muscular dystrophy, and cancer.

7. Hydrogen ion concentration measured as pH is responsible for the acidic or base nature of the compound. The lower the pH value, the higher concentration of hydrogen ions in the solution.

The Present Hypothesis

Our first thought that vascular calcification might be a result of acidosis occurred in 2006, during the development of the Acidity Theory of Atherosclerosis

I published the Portuguese version of "The Acidity Theory in Atherosclerosis – New Evidences" in 2011 and an English version in 2012, in which I cited some studies linking osteoporosis to atherosclerosis, as follows:

Although the prevalence of both atherosclerosis and osteoporosis increase with age, various and accumulating evidence indicates, since the initial studies, a more direct relationship between these two disorders. Confirming this association, many recent studies have shown an increase in carotid intima-media thickness, a marker for atherosclerosis, among women as they develop osteoporosis.

Hip fracture, a frequent complication of osteoporosis, is two to five times more common in patients with heart disease than in those with no history of cardiovascular problems. Other studies have shown that bisphosphonates not only decreased the progression of osteoporosis, but also inhibited the development of atherosclerosis, in addition to reducing total mortality. In that regard, it is important to note that bisphosphonates also reduce the production of lactic acid, which further supports the hypothesis that lactic acidosis may be involved in the etiology and pathogenesis of coronary heart disease. This also substantiates the role of stress in coronary atherosclerosis, since chronic stress increases lactate.

I also referred to the 1968 postulation by A. Wachman and D.S. Bernstein that bone mineral from skeletal dissolution functioned as a buffer base to neutralize the fixed acid load imposed by an "acid ash" diet as we age, which would lead to osteoporosis. However, the dietary acid-base hypothesis of bone loss remains controversial.

More recently, a 2018 study proposed that coronary artery calcification, previously thought to be a passive, degenerative and quiescent process, should now be viewed as an active process associated with increasing atherosclerosis by mechanisms similar to those involved in bone development. Another 2018 study also suggested that coronary arterial calcification shares some features with skeletal bone formation, including chondrocyte and osteoblast differentiation, mineralization, and bone matrix deposition and resorption. It is not unlikely that other mechanisms may be involved.

A few months later we consolidated all the necessary facts to present the hypothesis that increased lactic acid/lactate production might be responsible for coronary artery calcification. This theory was presented at the March 2019 "Fifth International Congress for Advanced Cardiac Sciences (King of Organs)" Conference in Saudi Arabia. In this presentation, we also shared the belief that acidosis was the culprit for bone loss with age, but that the triggering source was not the "acid ash" diet proposed by Wachman and Bernstein, but acidosis, especially lactic acidosis. In addition, acidosis is a causative factor in coronary artery calcification, based on our 2006 acidity theory of atherosclerosis. In the 2019 "King of Organs" Conference, I discussed the numerous risk factors that are associated with lactic acidosis, osteoporosis and coronary artery calcification, such as:

- Age

- Diabetes

- Hypertension

- Smoking

- Chronic Kidney Disease

- High Carbohydrate Diets

- Rheumatoid Arthritis

- Air Pollution

I also discussed diseases associated with lactic acidosis and coronary artery calcification, including stroke, cancer and myocardial infarction as well as drugs like statins, warfarin and metformin that are associated with this, as well as osteoporosis in some instances.

Some Highlights and Conclusions

1) Increased brain lactate is a hallmark of aging. In the aging skeleton, bone volume and mass declines in both sexes and in people of all ethnic backgrounds and is often associated with osteoporosis and an increased risk of fracture.

2) Elevated circulating lactate is a common occurrence in diabetic patients and this finding suggests that it may contribute to the increased prevalence of vascular calcification in this population.

3) High levels of sugar-sweetened carbonated beverage consumption may be associated with a higher prevalence and degree of coronary artery calcium (CAC) in asymptomatic adults without a history of cardiovascular disease, cancer, or diabetes.

4) Diets low in carbohydrate and high in fat and/or protein, regardless of the sources of protein and fat, were not associated with higher levels of CAC, a validated predictor of cardiovascular events, in this large multi-ethnic cohort.

5) A 2016 study found that statin intake in subjects with an LDL cholesterol equal to or greater than 115 milligrams per decilitre, was associated with lower coronary artery calcification progression than statin intake in subjects with LDL cholesterol levels below 115 mg/dL. But as the authors of the guidelines tend to be selective in choosing their references, they tend to neglect this and similar studies. The guidelines, built on cherry picked data, suggest that

individuals with an optimal LDL-C at or below 100 mg/dL have lower rates of heart disease and stroke, and some claim that LDL-C should be lowered as much as possible. This could pose a perplexing problem for physicians when prescribing statins. The acidity theory of atherosclerosis may be helpful in this regard, because of the following findings: a) Lowering pH augments the oxidation of low-density lipoprotein (LDL) by releasing iron and copper radicals and decreasing anti-oxidant defences, and b) LDL oxidation occurs within lysosomes in macrophages of atherosclerotic lesions rather than the surrounding interstitial fluid. Most importantly, studies have shown that this oxidative process can be promoted by an acidic pH, and is inhibited by chloroquine, which increases lysosome pH.

6) Acidosis is a hallmark of stroke. The presence and severity of coronary artery calcification is an independent predictor of future stroke events in the general population.

7) Acidosis is a hallmark of cancer. A recent study has demonstrated an increase in the incidence of coronary artery calcification over time in individuals with cancer compared with non-cancer controls. This relationship persisted even when other risk factors for atherosclerosis were excluded. A subsequent study revealed that cancer chemotherapy can also worsen CAC.

Carlos ETB Monteiro

Independent Researcher and Scientist
President, Infarct Combat Project (www.infarctcombat.org)
Fellow, The American Institute of Stress (www.stress.org)

Suggested Reading

1. Schade DS.1982. The role of catecholamines in metabolic acidosis. Ciba Found Symp;87:235-53 at https://www.ncbi.nlm.nih.gov/pubmed/6918290

2. Cori CF and Cori GT. The mechanism of epinephrine action IV: The influence of epinephrine on lactic acid production and blood sugar utilization. J Biol Chem 84: 683 – 698. 1929. Full text at http://www.jbc.org/content/84/2/683.full.pdf+html

3. Monteiro CETB. Stress as Cause of Heart Attacks – The Myogenic Theory. Published at the Journal Wise Traditions in Food, Farming, and the Healing Arts, Fall 2014. Reproduced by Positive Health Online, Edition 222 – May 2015 at https://bit.ly/2JPr5FC

4. Monteiro CETB. Stress as the Inductive Factor for Increased Lactate Production: The Evolutionary Path to Carcinogenesis. Positive Health Online, Edition 241, October 2017 at https://bit.ly/2Yj6b5d

5. Monteiro CETB. Monteiro CETB. Intense Stress Leading to Raised Production and Accumulation of Lactate in Brain Ischemia – The Ultimate Cause of Acute Stroke: Mechanism, Risk Factors and Therapeutics. Published in Positive Health Online, Edition 247, July 2018 at https://bit.ly/2YiGNwj

6. Monteiro CETB. Autonomic Dysfunction and Increased Lactate Production with Accumulation in the Body: The Key Factors for the Development of Rheumatoid Arthritis. Positive Health Online, Issue 252 - February 2019 at https://bit.ly/2wQSE90

7. Monteiro CETB. Acidic environment evoked by chronic stress: A novel mechanism to explain atherogenesis. Available from Infarct Combat Project, January 28, 2008 at http://www.infarctcombat.org/AcidityTheory.pdf

8. Monteiro CETB. Acidity Theory of Atherosclerosis – History, Pathophysiology, Therapeutics and Risk Factors – A Mini Review. Positive Health Online, Edition 226, November 2015 at http://goo.gl/AejGAV;

9. Monteiro CETB. Acidity Theory of Atherosclerosis: New Evidences, 2012 at https://www.amazon.com/Acidity-Theory-Atherosclerosis-New-Evidences/dp/1469934760;

10. Monteiro CETB. Stress as Cause of Atherosclerosis – The Acidity Theory, pp. 205-224 in Rosch, PJ ed. Fat and Cholesterol Don't Cause Heart Attacks and Statins Are Not The Solution. 2016 at https://www.amazon.com/Cholesterol-Cause-Attacks-Statins-Solution/dp/190779753X/

11. Mencken H L. Exeunt Omnes. Smart Set;1919 60: 138–145.

12. Wachman A, Bernstein DS. Diet and osteoporosis. *Lancet.* 1968;1:958–9 at https://www.sciencedirect.com/science/article/pii/S0140673668909082

The Crucial Role of Stress In Coronary Heart Disease

Paul J. Rosch MD

Stress, Emotions and The Heart in Ancient Cultures

The important contribution of emotions, personality and temperament to heart disease has been recognized since antiquity. Early cultures viewed the heart as the central organ that nourished the rest of the body. However, it had different meanings and connotations, since it was considered to be the seat of such varied emotions as fear, love, sorrow, courage, joy, anger and hatred. In some instances, the heart also depicted personality and the ability to distinguish right from wrong, or conscience. "Heart" occurs over one thousand times in the Bible, making it the most frequent anthropological term.

For example, Abraham offers his weary guests food so that they might *"sustain their hearts"* (Genesis 18:5). The heart thinks (Matt 9:4, Mark 2:8), remembers, reflects, and meditates (Psalm 77:5-6, Luke 2:19). Solomon's comprehensive knowledge of flora and fauna is described as his *"breadth of heart"* (1 Kings 4:29). Just as the eyes were meant to see and the ears to hear, the heart is meant to understand, to discern, to give insight. Around 200 B.C., Alexandrian Jewish scribes translated into Greek the Hebrew text of Proverbs 2:10, *"wisdom will enter your heart"* by *"wisdom will come into your understanding"* because to them it meant the same thing. When a person lacks insight the Hebrew views it as a *"lack of heart."*

The ancient Chinese thought the heart (*xin*) was the source of happiness and the hub of all other emotions. It was also the seat of wisdom and moral values that made it a *"fountainhead of happiness"*. Since *xin* could also mean mind, this holistic perspective viewed the heart as the center of both emotions and thought.[1] A Hindu scripture dating from 200 to 400 B.C, describes the *Paramatma* as the supreme soul that resides in the heart of every living entity.[2] The heart chakra was also the location of complex emotions like compassion, tenderness and unconditional love.[3]

The Greeks and Romans also believed the heart was the seat of the mind as well as the soul. The fourth century B. C. Greek philosopher Aristotle identified the heart as the most important organ of the body, as it was the first to form based on his observations of chick embryos. He described it as a three-chambered organ that was the seat of intelligence, motion, sensation and vitality in the body. Since it was hot and dry, he thought other organs like the brain and lungs existed primarily to cool the heart. These views were reiterated by the 2nd century Roman physician Galen, who wrote *"The heart is, as it were, the hearthstone and source of the innate heat by which the animal is governed."*[4] It was also the organ most closely related to the soul. However, Galen did not agree with Aristotle's claim that the heart is the origin of the nerves, and thought the liver was more important, since this was where blood and the other humors (yellow bile, black bile, and phlegm) were made. Galen was the most renowned physician of his era, and his views were considered to be irrefutable, especially since they were endorsed and promulgated by the Vatican. Anyone who contradicted or disputed Galen could be punished for heresy, which is why he has often been referred to as "The Medical Pope of the Middle Ages".

Medieval physicians had difficulty in reconciling the differing opinions of Aristotle and Galen, and Ibn Sina, an Arabic physician and philosopher, tried to incorporate them in his 1025 *Qanun fi al-Tibb* (The Canon of Medicine) as follows, *"The heart is the root of all faculties and gives the faculties of nutrition, life, apprehension, and movement to several other members."* He believed that heart produced breath, the *"vital power or innate heat"* within the body and was also an intelligent organ that controlled and directed all others. He identified the pulse as *"a movement in the heart and arteries which takes the form of alternate expansion and contraction, whereby the breath becomes subjected to the influence of the air inspired."* Ibn Sina, often referred to as Avicenna, his Latinized name, wrote over 400 tracts or books, but his 14-volume medical encyclopedia *Qanun* was the most important, since it contained over one million words of text that was divided and subdivided to cover every conceivable aspect of medical practice. A Latin translation of the *Qanun (Canon Medicinae)* appeared in Europe in the 11th century, quickly followed by others, and its 1593 publication in Rome made it one of the first Arabic books to be printed. It was reprinted in Europe more than thirty-five times during the 15th and 16th centuries alone, and from the 12th to 18th century, the *Qanun* was the most important medical text in the world because of its comprehensiveness and systematic arrangement.[5] It is believed to have influenced Leonardo Da Vinci, and Sir William Osler wrote, "*The Qanun has remained a medical bible for a longer time than any other work.*"

This Muslim belief that mind and soul were located in the heart was likely influenced by the early Egyptians, who regarded the heart, rather than the brain, as the source of wisdom, emotions, memory, and personality. Papyri written prior to 1500 B.C. describe the metu, channels emanating from the heart, which disseminated energy and information to other parts of the body by delivering not only blood, but air, nutrients, tears and saliva. Good health depended on the metu being clear and not blocked, much like an irrigation canal from the Nile that cannot deliver water when it is blocked. Similarly, most diseases were treated by attempting to dredge the metu, in an attempt to regulate, balance, and restore normal function, or remove noxious substances. These efforts started with the heart, which is why it was the only major organ not removed during mummification. The only function of the brain was thought to be to pass mucus to the nose, so it was discarded. To prevent the heart from providing damaging testimony during the final judgment, a scarab was often wrapped within the bandages containing inscriptions from the Book of the Dead, such as "*O my heart which I had upon earth, do not rise up against me as a witness in the presence of the lord of things; do not speak against me concerning what I have done, do not bring up anything against me in the presence of the great god of the West.*"[6] In Islamic medicine, both the Quran and Hadeeth emphasized the heart as the center for emotions, attitude and intellect. It is the heart that "*softens*" or "*hardens*". "*It is the hearts of the disbelievers that are blind, not their eyes*", and "*who have hearts that do not understand the Truth*". It was through the heart that Allah spoke, and his will was made known. Inshallah! (If Allah wills it).[7]

Stress, Emotions and The Heart in Western Medicine

It was also through Arabic translations that the West learned of Hellenic medicine, including the works of Galen and Hippocrates. Some highlights include:

Aulus Cornelius Celsus (30 B.C.) Roman physician and encyclopedist, *"Fear and anger, and any other state of the mind may often be apt to excite the pulse."*

William Harvey (1628) London physician who discovered how the blood circulates, *"Every affection of the mind that is attended either with pain or pleasure, hope or fear, is the cause of an agitation whose influence extends to the heart."*[8]

John Hunter (1793) English physician who elevated surgery from a mechanical trade to a medical specialty suffered from angina, and being a keen observer, told a friend *"My life is in the hands of any rascal who chooses to annoy and tease me"*, since he was fearful that *"some unpleasant dispute might occur"* at a forthcoming Board Meeting at St George's Hospital in London. This turned out to be quite prophetic, since the October 16, 1793 meeting was confrontational with heated discussions that rebuffed Hunter's views. According to onlookers, he *"immediately ceased speaking"* and left the room. Apparently unable to suppress the *"tumult of his passion"*, he had scarcely reached the privacy of an adjoining room when *"with a deep groan"* he fell lifeless into the arms of a colleague and was pronounced dead at the scene.[9] An autopsy performed by his brother-in-law, Everard Home identified the cause of death to be a diseased heart resulting from angina pectoris: the carotid arteries and their branches being *"thickened and ossified"* and the pericardium was unusually *"thick"*. Home concluded that Hunter's 65-year-old heart was *"unable to carry out its functions, whenever the actions were disturbed"*, either in *"consequence of bodily exertion or affections of the mind."*[10]

Jean-Nicholas Corvisart (1815) Napoleon's favorite physician, wrote that heart disease was due to the *"passions of the mind"* (which included anger, madness, fear, jealousy, terror, love, despair, joy, avarice, stupidity and ambition).[11]

Job Stress and Type A Coronary Prone Behavior

The relationship between job stress and illness was recognized over 300 years ago by Bernardo Ramazzini, who described in detail the

74

diseases of people engaged in 40 different kinds of work and urged his fellow physicians to question their patients about their occupations. While the major focus was on physical hazards such as *"sharp and acid particles"* in the air at certain work environments, he was well aware of the role of personal habits, behavior and psychosocial factors in causing illness and emphasized the importance of prevention.[12] Theodor von Dusch (1850), a German physician, first called attention to the fact that excessive involvement in work appeared to be the hallmark of people who developed coronary heart disease.[13]

Sir William Osler (1910), described the coronary prone individual as a *"keen, and ambitious man, the indicator of whose engines are set at 'full speed ahead.'"* He also wrote that he could make the presumptive diagnosis of angina based on the appearance, demeanor and behavior of the patient in the waiting room.[14] Flanders Dunbar, who introduced the term "psychosomatic" into American medicine,[15] characterized such individuals as being authoritarian with an intense drive to achieve unrealistic goals.[16] The Menningers (1936) suggested that heart attack patients tended to have strongly aggressive behavior.[17]

Fierce ambition and compulsiveness to achieve power and prestige were emphasized by subsequent investigators, and the rising incidence of coronary heart disease in England over the next two decades was attributed to increased job stress,[18] in addition to low social status.[19]

All of these 19th and 20th century physicians were describing various aspects of what is now called Type A behavior, a term coined by Meyer Friedman and Ray Rosenman in 1959.[20] Type A individuals are apt to be very competitive and are usually in a hurry, so they eat, talk, and do most other activities as quickly as possible. They generally try to do too many things at the same time, are frequently concerned with what they are going to do next and are often so preoccupied with work that they tend to have few other interests. Around the same time, Stewart Wolf independently noted that coronary disease was often due to the constant striving to achieve unrealistic goals, adding that even when successful, such individuals were unable to relax and enjoy the satisfaction of their labors. He called this the *"Sisyphus Syndrome"*, since in Greek mythology, Sisyphus was the king of Corinth, and the most cunning and immoral person imaginable. He boasted he was more clever and powerful than Zeus, and as a punishment, was banished to Hades, where he had to repeatedly roll a huge boulder to the top of a steep hill, only to have it roll back down to the base as soon as the summit was reached. Other Greek mythological portrayals of Hell also viewed it as a place of perpetual but fruitless labor. Stewart described individuals who were constantly preoccupied with work, even when it was not productive, as suffering from the Sisyphus syndrome, and demonstrated that they had a significantly increased risk for heart attacks.

It is important to emphasize that Rosenman and Friedman were cardiologists with no expertise in psychology. Psychiatrists and others had previously described various personality characteristics in patients who seemed to be prone to heart attacks but Rosenman and Friedman were not aware of this at the time. The careful observations that led to their Type A theory required an unusual combination of curiosity, diagnostic acumen and a biopsychosocial approach to the patient as a person, rather than someone with symptoms and signs that required treatment in a cookbook fashion.

Their primary interest was in cholesterol, since by 1950, although fat and cholesterol had long been fed to rabbits to produce vascular lesions, little was known about where plasma cholesterol came from or how it was metabolized. They also noted that this type of vascular plaque was quite different from that seen in patients with coronary artery disease. They obtained grants to investigate cholesterol metabolism in animals and subsequently delineated many fundamental aspects of this as well as the mechanisms underlying low and high plasma cholesterol respectively in hypothyroidism and hyperthyroidism, as well as what caused elevated lipids in patients with nephrosis. Around 1952, because of their growing interest in cholesterol, they obtained blood samples from private patients at every visit for (no-cost) accurate analyses at their research lab. They soon realized that their cholesterol levels were unrelated to diet or weight and that there were surprising fluctuations, and they pursued this in subsequent studies.

They later recognized and reported serious errors and omissions in papers by Keys and others about the contribution of diet to plasma cholesterol. The prevailing dogma, which still persists, was that coronary heart disease was due to an elevated cholesterol, which in turn resulted from increased dietary fat intake. Their observations and other data that Keys had ignored in reaching his conclusions did not support this and reinforced their belief that socioeconomic influences played a more important role in the increased incidence of coronary disease. Their perceptive office manager mentioned that in contrast to other patients, those with coronary disease were rarely late for appointments and preferred to sit in hard-upholstered chairs rather than softer ones or sofas. These chairs also had to be reupholstered far more frequently than others because the front edges quickly became worn out. They repeatedly looked at their watches, acted impatient when they had to wait, usually sat on the edges of waiting room chairs and tended to leap up when called to be examined.[21] Her astute observations were similar to those made by Sir William Osler, and more intensive scrutiny revealed the following characteristics:

- Self-imposed standards that are often unrealistically ambitious and pursued in an inflexible fashion.

- Associated with this is a need to maintain productivity in order to be respected, a sense of guilt while on vacation or relaxing, an unrelenting urge for recognition or power, and a competitive attitude that often creates challenges even when none exist.

- Certain thought and activity styles characterized by persistent vigilance and impulsiveness, usually resulting in the pursuit of several lines of thought or action simultaneously.

- Hyperactive responsiveness often manifested by a tendency to interrupt or finish a sentence in conversation, usually in dramatic fashion, by varying the speech, volume, and/or pitch, or by alternating rapid bursts of words with long pauses of hesitation for emphasis, indicating intensive thought. Type A persons often nod or mutter agreement or use short bursts of laughter to obliquely indicate to the speaker that the point being made has already been anticipated so that they can take over.

- Unsatisfactory interpersonal relationships due to the fact that Type As are usually self-centered, poor listeners, often have an attitude of bravado about their own superiority, and are much more easily angered, frustrated, or hostile if their wishes are not respected or their goals are not achieved.

- Increased muscular activity in the form of gestures, motions, and facial activities such as grimaces, gritting and grinding of the teeth, or tensing jaw muscles. Often there is frequent clenching of the fist or perhaps pounding with a fist to emphasize a point. Fidgeting, tapping the feet, leg shaking, or playing with a pencil in some rhythmic fashion are also common.

- Irregular or unusual breathing patterns with frequent sighing, produced by inhaling more air than needed during speaking and then releasing it during the middle or end of a sentence for emphasis.

- Type As tend to be very competitive and are usually in a hurry, so they eat, talk, and do most other activities as quickly as possible.

- They generally try to do too many things at the same time, are frequently concerned with what they are going to do next and are often so preoccupied with work that they tend to have few other interests.[22]

Type A has been acknowledged by the NIH to be as powerful a predictor of heart attacks as cholesterol or any other risk factor.[23]

Why Stress is Much More Important than Lipids

- Stress increases the original Framingham standard risk factors of cholesterol, smoking and hypertension, as well as diabetes, obesity and hs-CRP.

- Stressful life change events, depression, anxiety, Type A behavior and hostility have all been linked to an increased incidence of coronary events.

- Stress causes coronary vasoconstriction as well as an increase in platelet stickiness and aggregation that promote clot formation.

- Stress increases levels of homocysteine and lactic acid, as well as fibrinogen and other coagulation factors that contribute to coronary heart disease.

- Stress causes deep abdominal fat deposits, which secrete inflammatory cytokines that lead to insulin resistance and the cardiovascular complications of metabolic syndrome.

- The $150 million ($800 million today) 10-year MRFIT study found no benefit in reducing cholesterol, smoking and hypertension. In contrast, two other studies during the same period were halted prematurely since they were so successful in preventing heart attacks. One was behavioral modification to reduce Type A traits, and the other was treatment with Inderal, a drug that blocks the effects of stress hormones like cortisol.

- The INTERHEART study done in six continents to determine causes of CHD, found that psychosocial stress was a major factor.

- Stress causes atrial fibrillation, the most common sustained arrhythmia, as well as ventricular fibrillation, the leading cause of sudden death.

- Over half of patients with paroxysmal atrial fibrillation attribute the onset of an attack with antecedent stress.

- Stress can precipitate and worsen congestive heart failure.

- Severe stress can cause a myocardial infarction in the absence of any coronary occlusion due to direct myocardial damage from the secretion of norepinephrine at nerve endings and has been seen in healthy teenagers with no heart disease.

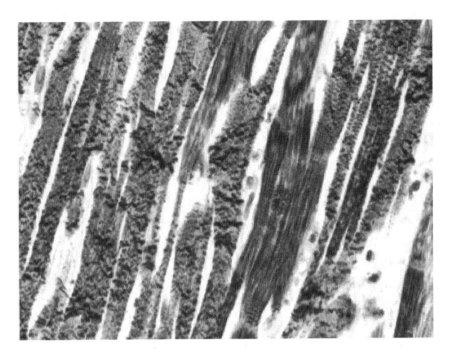

FIGURE 1 **Contraction band necrosis**[24]

This produces a characteristic contraction band necrosis called coagulative myocytolysis, as illustrated above. This necrosis can be seen in sudden death following severe stress in healthy animals and people and has been reported in patients with a pheochromocytoma, an adrenal medullary tumor that secretes excess catecholamines. It can also be induced in animals by giving intravenous norepinephrine. As can be seen this lesion has none of the white cell infiltration or signs of inflammation that are usually seen in acute myocardial infarctions due to coronary heart disease.

Other Effects of Acute Stress on The Heart

Stress related left ventricular apical ballooning is referred to as "*Takotsubo Cardiomyopathy*," since it resembles the tako-tsubo fishing pot with a narrow neck and wide base the Japanese use to trap octopuses in Japan. This "*myocardial stunning*" is due to left ventricular contractile dysfunction during systole, as shown to the left. It usually occurs in post-menopausal women with no history of coronary heart disease, who present severe chest pain and shortness of breath.

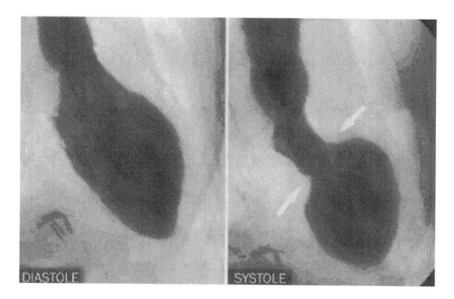

FIGURE 2 **Takotsubo Cardiomyopathy**[25]

Although there is no evidence of coronary occlusion, ECGs show marked ischemic changes similar to those seen in acute myocardial infarction. However, these usually spontaneously return to normal within 48 to 72 hours and patients return home in a week. The cause is unknown, but because it often occurs after the sudden loss of a loved one, it has been nicknamed *"The Broken Heart Syndrome"*.

One of the most compelling and convincing illustrations of the effects of acute stress on the heart comes from Holter (ambulatory) ECG recordings in patients suddenly exposed to a severe earthquake. In the 1999 Taiwan earthquake, there were 12 such patients, and a review of their tracings showed a marked increase in heart rate up to 160 beats/min when the quake occurred. In addition, there was a change in heart rate variability with a lowering of high frequency and an increase in low frequency variability, suggesting increased sympathetic and subdued parasympathetic nervous system responses. These changes were reduced in patients taking beta-blockers.[26]

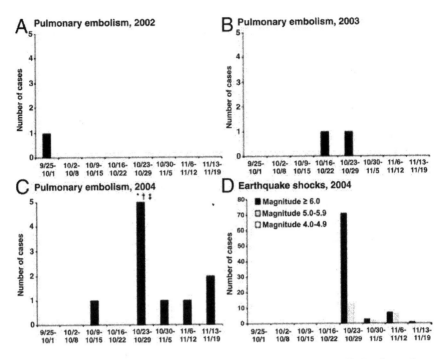

FIGURE 3 Incidence of Pulmonary Embolism Associated With Earthquakes

Patients with pulmonary embolism (A to C) and shock in the 2004 Niigata-Chuetsu earthquake (D). Pulmonary embolism increased after the earthquake compared with the prior 4 weeks and the corresponding 8 weeks in 2002 and 2003. The number of shocks was obtained from the official records of the Niigata-Chuetsu earthquake by Japan Meteorological. $p <$ 0.001 versus prior 4 weeks in 2004 or corresponding 8 weeks in 2002 and 2003.[27]

The number of cardiovascular deaths in the January 17, 1994 Northridge, California earthquake skyrocketed on that date, compared to such deaths on January 17 in the three previous years. In the 1995 Japanese Hanshin-Awaji earthquake, blood pressure also increased, and blood pressures failed to show the usual nocturnal drop. There was a rise in blood viscosity, and blood clotting was accelerated due to increased fibrinogen, von Willebrand factor and other contributors to coagulation. This quickened blood clotting is important since it had other unanticipated adverse effects. In 2004, Central Nigata, Japan, suffered 3 strong earthquakes and 90 aftershocks in the ensuing week. One hundred thousand residents were evacuated from their homes,

82

and many spent nights sleeping in their cars that resulted in relative immobilization in a cramped position for prolonged periods of time. As will be seen, this resulted in a dramatic increase in pulmonary embolism that might have been due to impaired circulation in the lower extremities. This, along with the associated psychological stress, promoted the development of venous clots that broke off and traveled to the lungs to cause pulmonary emboli, as illustrated below.

The Effects of Chronic Stress on The Heart

- Chronic stress due to depression, job pressures, discrimination, caregiving, financial or family problems is associated with increased risk of death due to heart attack and stroke.

- With respect to stressful life change events, loss of a spouse is at the top of the list, so it is not surprising that up to 20 percent of their mates will die within 12 to 18 months, often from a heart attack, especially if they are elderly.[28, 29]

- In one review of chronic work related stress, meeting future deadlines was associated with a six-fold increase in myocardial infarction.[30]

- Other studies show that chronic job stress is associated with two to three times higher rate of coronary events in employees who perceive they have little control over their work demands.[31]

- Caring for a sick spouse or relative with Alzheimer's or some other chronic illness at home nearly doubles heart disease death rates.[32]

- In women with established coronary disease, those complaining of increased marital stress were three times more apt to have experienced recurrent events than controls with little marital discord.[33] Such events can be significantly lowered by developing good coping skills, as well as stress reduction techniques.[34]

One effective technique is meditation, as illustrated below.

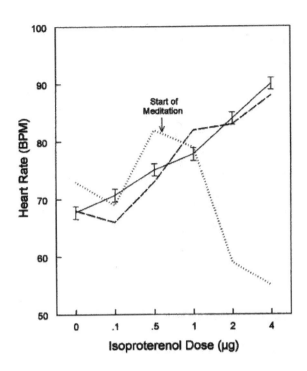

FIGURE 4 **Effect of Meditation on Heart Rate Response to Infused Isoproterenol[35]**

Chronotropic responses to isoproterenol. (Solid line) Mean ± standard error response to isoproterenol in 93 women; (dotted line) patient's response while meditating; (dashed line), patient's response while instructed not to meditate.

Isoproterenol is used to treat Adam-Stokes syncope, cardiac arrest, heart block, and severe asthmatic attacks. It is a beta adrenergic agonist that increases heart rate. This effect can be reduced by beta blockers like Inderal, but, as shown to the left, meditation also causes a prompt and dramatic reduction. Meditation, yoga and beta blockers can also reduce stress induced hypertension. The beneficial cardiovascular effects of regular aerobic exercise like jogging as well as yoga and progressive muscular relaxation have also been attributed to lowering stress levels. When any of these are practiced on a routine basis, there is usually a lowering of elevated blood pressure that reduces the risk for stroke, as well as coronary events.

Other Adverse Effects of Chronic Stress

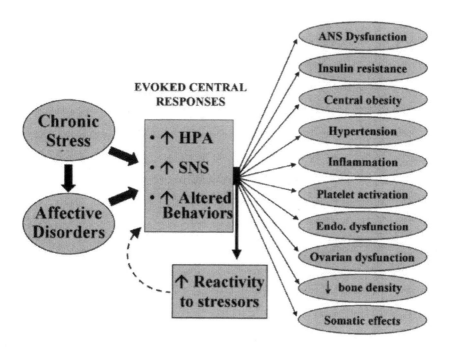

FIGURE 5 **How Chronic Stress Causes Cardiovascular and Other Adverse Effects**

As shown above, chronic stress can contribute to coronary atherosclerosis by varied influences, including the HPA (hypothalamic-pituitary axis), SNS (sympathetic nervous system) and ANS (autonomic nervous system). Chronic stress also influences behaviors like smoking, excess alcoholic intake, chocolate and other comfort foods rich in sugar that are much more likely to contribute to cardiovascular disease than an elevated cholesterol or LDL.[36]

But it's much more complicated when you consider the combined effects of repetitive acute as well as persistent stress and their multiple interactions. Repeated episodes of acute stress or chronic stress can initiate and promote the atherosclerotic process. Stress induces cytokines, which, together with the major stress hormones corticosteroids and catecholamines, induce acute phase proteins (APPs) in the liver. Recurrent stress or chronic stress, with changes in blood flow and blood pressure, causes endothelial damage and adhesion of platelets. Cytokines, corticosteroids, and other factors induce adhesion molecules at sites of endothelial change, to which recruited monocytes and lymphocytes adhere and translocate to the arterial wall. Repeated or chronic stress, together with the acute phase reactants, promotes progression of the inflammatory response, with activation of macrophages and ensuing free radical formation, modification of lipids, foam cell formation, and activation of thrombotic events resulting in stable or unstable plaques. Elevation of homocysteine, which may also be induced by stress, would contribute to endothelial damage, platelet activation, thrombosis, the inflammatory process, smooth muscle cell hyperplasia, and proteolytic enzyme formation. Elevated homocysteine would augment lipid oxidation by oxidant stress and foam cell formation from LDL–homocysteine aggregates. Stress-induced activation of intimal mast cells by a neurogenic inflammatory process would also likely contribute to the inflammation, as illustrated below in Figure 6.[37]

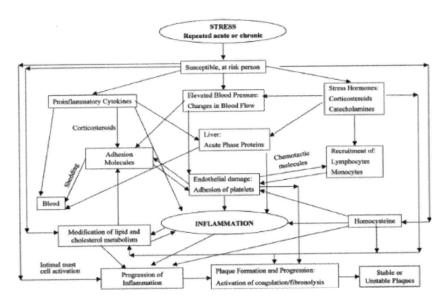

FIGURE 6 **How Acute And Chronic Stress Contribute To Inflammation And Atherosclerotic Plaque**

The Amygdala and Susceptibility to Stress

The amygdala is a cluster of nuclei located deep in the temporal lobes that are involved in processing emotions such as fear, anger, anxiety and pleasure. They have close connections with the hippocampus and hypothalamus, as well as the cerebral cortex and brainstem. Sophisticated imaging studies confirm that increased amygdala activity is associated with increased risk of a cardiovascular event because it stimulates the HPA axis as well as the sympathetic nervous system, resulting in an increase in cortisol and catecholamines. It also increases atherosclerotic inflammation in arteries by activating the bone marrow to release cytokines that promote atherosclerotic inflammation and its atherothrombotic consequences as shown to the left. There may be other pathways as well and delineating these may lead to innovative ways to prevent stress induced cardiovascular disease by inhibiting excess amygdala activity or blocking a key component of one of its pathways.[38, 39]

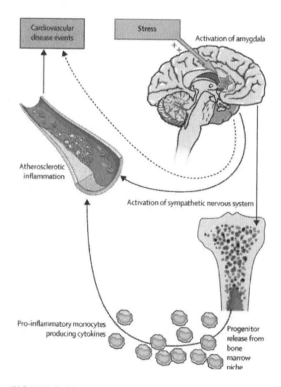

FIGURE 7 Stress and Atherosclerotic Inflammation[39]

In addition to such specially designed pharmaceuticals, energy therapies such as electromagnetic stimulation may be superior. This has already been demonstrated with rTMS (repetitive transcranial magnetic stimulation) that significantly and promptly improves drug resistant depression.[40] Vagus nerve stimulation, which activates the cholinergic anti-inflammatory pathway, is superior to and tolerated better than drugs in autoimmune disorders like rheumatoid arthritis.[41] The future for novel, more effective and safer stress reduction therapies looks bright, and is on the horizon.

Paul J. Rosch, MD

FACP Clinical Professor of Medicine and Psychiatry, New York Medical College, Valhalla, NY, USA and Chairman of the Board, The American Institute of Stress, Weatherford TX, USA

References

1. Yu N. The Chinese HEART in a Cognitive Perspective: Culture, Body, and Language. 2009; De Gruyter Mouton, Berlin.

2. Robinson CA. Interpretations of the Bhagavad-Gita and Images of the Hindu tradition. 2014; Taylor & Francis. Boca Raton, pp. viii–ix.

3. Minor RN. Modern Indian Interpreters of the Bhagavad Gita. 1986; State University of New York Press, Albany.

4. Galen C. On the Usefulness of the Parts of the Body. Trans. Margaret Tallmadge 1968; Cornell University Press, Ithaca.

5. Chamsi-Pasha MAR, Chamsi-Pasha H. Avicenna's contribution to cardiology. Avicenna J Med. 2014; 4: 9–12.

6. Kemp, B. How to Read the Egyptian Book of the Dead. 2007 Granta Publications. New York, pp. 112–113.

7. Faulkner, RO The Ancient Egyptian Book of the Dead. 1972; University of Texas Press, Austin.

8. Harvey W. Exercitatio anatomica de motu cordis et sanguinis in animalibus. 1628; Sumptibus Gulielmi Fizer, Francofurti.

9. Palmer JF. The Works of John Hunter. 1835; Rees, Orme, Browne, Green and Longman, London p. 131.

10. Brian L. The Spasms of John Hunter: A New Interpretation. Medical History. 1973;17:70–75.

11. Corvisart JN., An essay on the organic diseases and lesions of the heart and great vessels, 1806 trans. Jacob Gates 1962; Hafner, New York, pp. 27.

12. Ramazzini B. Translation of the Latin text of De Morbus Artificum Diatriba of 1713 by the NY Academy of Medicine 1964; Havner Press, New York.

13. Von Dusch T. Lehrbuch der Herzkrankeiten. 1868; Verlag von Wilhelm Engelman, Leipzig.

14. Osler W. The Lumleian Lectures on Angina Pectoris. *Lancet* 1910; i: 697–702 and 838–844.

15. Dunbar HF. Emotions And Bodily Changes. A Survey of Literature on Psychosomatic Interrelationships. Columbia University Press, New York.

16. Dunbar HF. Psychosomatic Diagnosis 1943; Hoeber, New York.

17. Menninger KA, Menninger WC. Psychoanalytic observations in cardiac disorders. Am Heart J. 1936; 11:10-21.

18. Kuper H, Marmot M. Job strain, job demands, decision latitude, and risk of coronary heart disease within the Whitehall II study. Journal of Epidemiology and Community Health. 2003; 57 (2): 147–153.

19. Marmot MG, Rose G, Shipley M. Hamilton P. Employment grade and coronary heart disease in British civil servants. Journal of Epidemiology and Community Health. 1978; 32 (4): 244 – 249.

20. Friedman, M, Rosenman, RH. Association of specific overt behavior patterns with blood and cardiovascular findings: Blood cholesterol level, blood clotting time, incidence of arcus senilis and clinical coronary artery disease. JAMA 1959 169: 1286-1296

21. Friedman M, Rosenman RH. Type A Behavior and Your Heart. 1974; Knopf, New York.

22. Rosch, PJ. Stress and Cardiovascular Disease. Comprehensive Therapy 1983; 9:6-13.

23. Review Panel on Coronary-Prone Behavior and Coronary Heart Disease: A critical review. Circulation. 1981; 63:1199-1215.

24. https://commons.wikimedia.org/

25. Sharkey SW, Lesser JR, Zenovich AG, *et al.* Acute reversible cardiomyopathy provoked by stress in women from the United States. Circulation. 2005; 111(4):472– 479.

26. Dimsdale JE. Psychological Stress and Cardiovascular Disease. J Am Coll Cardiol 2008;51:1237–46.

27. Watanabe H, Kodama M, Tanabe N, *et al.* Impact of earthquakes on risk for pulmonary embolism. Int J Cardiol 2008;129(1):152-4.

28. Carey IM, Shah SM, DeWilde S, Harris T, Victor CR, Cook DG. Increased Risk of Acute Cardiovascular Events After Partner Bereavement: A Matched Cohort Study. JAMA Intern Med. 2014;174(4):598–605.

29. Stroebe M, Schut H, Stroebe W. Health outcomes of bereavement. *Lancet.* 2007;370:1960-1973.

30. Chandola R, Britton A, Brunner E, *et al.* Work stress and coronary heart disease: what are the mechanisms? Eur Heart J. 2008; 29:640-648.

31. Jacob L, Kostev K. Conflicts at work are associated with a higher risk of cardiovascular disease. Ger Med Sci, 2017 Apr26; 15: Doc 08.

32. Ho A, Collins S, Davis K, Doty M. A Look at Working-Age Caregivers Roles, Health Concerns, and Need for Support 2008: The Commonwealth Fund, New York.

33. Orth-Gomer, K, Wamala SP, Horsten M, *et al.* Marital stress worsens prognosis in women with coronary heart disease: The Stockholm Female Coronary Risk Study. JAMA 2000; 284:3008-3014.

34. Orth-Gomer K, Schneiderman N, Wang HX, *et al.* Stress Reduction Prolongs Life in Women With Coronary Disease. The Stockholm Women's Intervention Trial for Coronary Heart Disease. Circulation: Cardiovascular Quality and Outcomes. 2009; 2:25–32.

35. Dimsdale JE, Mills PJ. An unanticipated effect of meditation on cardiovascular pharmacology and physiology. Am J Cardiol 2002; 90:908-9.

36. Rozanski A, Blumenthal JA, Kaplan J. Impact of psychological factors on the pathogenesis of cardiovascular disease and implications for therapy. Circulation.1999;99:2192-2217.

37. Vale S. Psychosocial stress and cardiovascular diseases. Postgraduate Medical Journal 2005;81:429-435.

38. Roozendaal B. McEwen BS, Chattarji S. Stress, memory and the amygdala. Nature Reviews Neuroscience. 2009; 10:423-433.

39. Tawakol A, Ishai A, Takx RA, Figueroa AL, Ali A, Kaiser Y, *et al.* Relation between resting amygdalar activity and cardiovascular events: a longitudinal and cohort study. *Lancet.* 2017; 389:834–45.

40. George MS, Short EB, Kerns S. *et al.* Repetitive Transcranial Magnetic Stimulation for Depression and Other Indications. In Rosch PJ ed. Bioelectromagnetic and Subtle Energy Medicine. 2014; pp 169-188; CRC Press, Boca Raton.

41. Koopman FA, Chavan S, Miljko *et al.* Vagus nerve stimulation inhibits cytokine production and attenuates disease severity in rheumatoid arthritis. Proceedings of the National Academy of Sciences. 2016; 113(29):605-635.

Infections May Cause Atherosclerosis and Coronary Heart Disease

Uffe Ravnskov MD PhD

It is commonly believed that high LDL-cholesterol interferes with the function of the endothelium (the inner layer of the arterial wall), which allows it to infiltrate the artery wall, where it is subsequently oxidized by macrophages (a type of white blood cells) and that it is this reaction which causes inflammation.

However, the hypothesis that high LDL-cholesterol causes endothelial dysfunction is unlikely, since in a study of patients with coronary heart disease symptoms, Reis and co-workers[1] found no association between LDL-cholesterol blood levels and the degree of endothelial dysfunction. The arteries of those with low LDL-cholesterol malfunctioned just as much as the arteries of those with high LDL-cholesterol. It is true that inflammation of the arterial wall is associated with increased atherosclerosis but the notion that it causes atherosclerosis is just as wrong as the erroneous belief that the culprit is an elevated cholesterol. If inflammation was the cause of atherosclerosis, then anti-inflammatory drugs should be beneficial by decreasing the risk, but it is just the opposite. A recent article in the *British Medical Journal*, which included almost half a million individuals,[2] found a significant increase in NSAID (non-steroid anti-inflammatory drug) treatment in the 61,460 who suffered an acute myocardial infarction. Taking any dose of NSAIDs for a week, a month, or more than a month was associated with an increased risk of myocardial infarction. The higher the dose, the higher the risk.

That such drugs are dangerous is also evident from the Vioxx fiasco. Vioxx (rofecoxib), an anti-inflammatory drug, was marketed by Merck & Co. in 1999 to treat migraine, dysmenorrhea, acute pain conditions and all kinds of joint disease. Five years later it was withdrawn from the market because it was evident that Vioxx increased the risk of coronary disease. It appeared that Merck had withheld this information from doctors and patients for over five years resulting in between 88,000 and 140,000 cases of serious heart disease, many of which were fatal. This scandal resulted in fines of approximately one billion dollars.

Inflammation is the body's normal response to irritation or injury, but most researchers are not aware that infections may be an important cause of arterial inflammation. More than one hundred years ago, bacteria and viruses were considered as the cause of atherosclerosis and cardiovascular disease. One reason for this was that people who died from typhoid fever were more atherosclerotic than normal, as were the radial arteries of those who survived. More recent studies from all over the world provide additional support for the role of infections.

A British analysis of 14 years of data from 1.2 million hospital records found that patients admitted with a urinary tract or pulmonary infection had a 40 percent greater chance of a heart attack, while stroke risk was increased by 150 percent. Those suffering such infections were three times as likely to die if they had coronary heart disease and almost twice as likely to die if they had a stroke.

The effects of infection were comparable to the increased risk associated with diabetes, hypertension, or high cholesterol, and greater than obesity.

A U.S. study that examined a registry of patients tracked over multiple years in four U.S. cities, reviewed the records of 1,312 patients who had a heart attack or other coronary event, and 727 other patients who had an ischemic stroke due to a blood clot. Of the heart disease patients, 37 percent had some type of infection within the previous three months, and for stroke patients, it was nearly 30 percent.[3]

Periodontal disease has been associated with coronary heart disease, and in an Italian trial of 35 healthy people with periodontitis, researchers succeeded in lowering the thickness of the arterial wall significantly by treating the infection,[4] whereas no statins have ever accomplished this.

In a Swedish study of 28 children with an infectious disease, researchers reported that compared to healthy children, the arteries of those who died from the infection were narrowed and that the arterial walls of those who survived were thickened.[5] It is also well-known that acute myocardial infarction patients often have fever, an elevated sedimentation rate and other laboratory changes seen in infections, and in severe cases, they may have sepsis (bacteria in the blood).

There is also experimental support for the infection hypothesis. For instance, early atherosclerosis can be produced in chickens by infecting them with herpes virus[6] and in mice by infecting them with various types of bacteria.[7] In a Danish minipig experiment, researchers produced signs of early atherosclerosis by infecting them with bacteria and/or viruses.[8] The worst changes were seen in minipigs infected with both bacteria and virus, as well as those with the lowest cholesterol levels.

The latter is an obvious contradiction to the general view about cholesterol. One explanation may be that the lipoproteins (molecules that transport cholesterol around in the blood) protect against infections by adhering to and inactivating all kinds of microorganisms and their toxic products.[9] Very few are aware of this. although it has been demonstrated in many ways by more than a dozen research groups. For example, most mice die if they are injected with bacterial toxins, but can survive if they have received an injection of purified human LDL (the lipoprotein which transports LDL-cholesterol) before the infection, and mice with familial hypercholesterolemia (inherited high cholesterol) have greater resistance to infections.

Conversely, many studies have also demonstrated that low cholesterol is associated with decreased resistance to infectious diseases. This finding has been explained by claiming that infections somehow lower cholesterol. However, in an American study, Iribarren and co-workers measured cholesterol in about 130,000 healthy youngsters.[10] Fifteen years later, they found that those whose cholesterol was the lowest at the start had been hospitalized more often due to an infectious disease than those with normal or high cholesterol. It is of course highly unlikely that a disease they had not yet suffered from should have been the cause of their low cholesterol. It is also relevant to mention the rare inborn disease named Smith-Lemly-Opitz syndrome. Children with this disease are born with a cholesterol which is just as low as that achieved with the new cholesterol-lowering drugs (the PCSK9-inhibitors). A common symptom of those who survive is frequent and serious infections and a high intake of cholesterol lowers the incidence and the severity of these infections.

A frequent and pertinent question is, how infections are able to cause atherosclerosis and cardiovascular disease. Along with Kilmer McCully,[9, 11] I have proposed a plausible explanation, since it has been shown that when microorganisms are covered with LDL-cholesterol, they aggregate and create large complexes in the blood. The size of these conglomerates can increase if the level of the amino acid homocysteine in the blood is too high, because homocysteine creates anti-LDL-antibodies. Because of the high extra-capillary pressure around the arteries, these clumps of bacteria may obstruct vasa vasorum, the capillaries that supply the arterial wall with oxygen and nutrients. Obstruction of vasa vasorum produces ischemia of the arterial wall; it becomes anoxic leading to an accumulation of toxic substances, foam cells (see below) and microorganisms creating a vulnerable plaque, a bubble in the arterial wall. In our view, this mechanism explains the presence of inflammation. In accordance, inflammation in atherosclerotic arteries is more pronounced in the adventitia (the outer layer of the arteries), the tissue where vasa vasorum are located; not in the intima; a strong contradiction to the common belief that inflammation starts in the intimal layer.

Most arterial blood clots are seen close to a vulnerable plaque. We think, as did William Osler over 100 years ago, that vulnerable plaque is a boil that can create a blood clot when it bursts. Several laboratory studies are in accord with this hypothesis. A common finding in atherosclerotic tissue are white blood cells filled with something that looks like foam and are called foam cells. But on closer scrutiny, the foam is actually clumping of bacteria. Laboratory experiments have shown that bacteria, viruses and their toxic products are able to convert white blood cells into foam cells if they are mixed with human LDL, and more than fifty different bacteria and virus types have been identified in atherosclerotic arteries, but not a single one in normal arteries.

It is a common belief that oxidized LDL-cholesterol is responsible for initiating atherosclerosis. However, when microorganisms are taken up by the macrophages, they are destroyed by oxidation. As they are covered with LDL-cholesterol, the reason why oxidized LDL-cholesterol is associated with cardiovascular disease is simply because LDL-cholesterol becomes oxidized as well. A high level of oxidized LDL-cholesterol is simply a sign of infection, and not the cause of atherosclerosis.

Uffe Ravnskov, MD PhD

Further reading

You can read more about our ideas in the following two papers, which I have published together with Kilmer McCully, he who discovered the strong association between homocysteine and atherosclerosis...

Ravnskov & McCully. "Vulnerable Plaque Formation from Obstruction of Vasa Vasorum by Homocysteinylated and Oxidized Lipoprotein Aggregates Complexed with Microbial Remnants and LDL Autoantibodies." Annals of Clinical & Laboratory Science, vol. 39, no. 1, 2009.

Ravnskov & McCully. "Infections May be Causal in the Pathogenesis of Atherosclerosis." The American Journal of the Medical Sciences, Volume 344, Number 5, November 2012.

... and in this paper, published with 15 international experts, which documents that high cholesterol is not the cause of cardiovascular disease:

Ravnskov *et al.* "LDL-C does not cause cardiovascular disease: a comprehensive review of the current literature." Expert Review of Clinical Pharmacology. 2018.

References

1. Reis SE, Holubkov R, Conrad-Smith AJ *et al.* Coronary microvascular dysfunction is highly prevalent in women with chest pain in the absence of coronary artery disease: results from the NHLBI WISE study. Am Heart J 2001;141:735-741.

2. Bally M, Dendukuri N, Rich B *et al.* Risk of acute myocardial infarction with NSAIDs in real world use: bayesian meta-analysis of individual patient data. BMJ 2017;357:j1909. doi1136/bmj.j1909.

3. Smeeth L, Thomas SL, Hall AJ, Hubbard R, Farrington P, Vallance P. Risk of myocardial infarction and stroke after acute infection or vaccination. NEJM 2004;351:2611-2618.

4. Piconi S, Trabattoni D, Luraghi C, *et al.* Treatment of periodontal disease results in improvements in endothelial dysfunction and reduction of the carotid intima-media thickness. FASEB J 2009;23:1196–204.

5. Liuba P, Persson J, Luoma J, *et al*. Acute infections in children are accompanied by oxidative modification of LDL and decrease of HDL cholesterol, and are followed by thickening of carotid intima-media. Eur Heart J 2003;24:515–21.

6. Fabricant CG, Fabricant J, Litrenta MM, *et al*. Virus-induced atherosclerosis. J Exp Med 1978;148:335–40.

7. Damy SB, Higuchi ML, Timenetsky J, *et al*. Mycoplasma pneumoniae and/or Chlamydophila pneumoniae inoculation causing different aggravations in cholesterol-induced atherosclerosis in apoE KO male mice. BMC Microbiol 2009;9:194–201.

8. Birck MM, Pesonen E, Odermarsky M, *et al*. Infection-induced coronary dysfunction and systemic inflammation in piglets are dampened in hypercholesterolemic milieu. Am J Physiol Heart Circ Physiol 2011;300:1595–601.

9. Ravnskov U, McCully KS. Vulnerable plaque formation from obstruction of vasa vasorum by homocysteinylated and oxidized lipoprotein aggregates complexed with microbial remnants and LDL autoantibodies. Ann Clin Lab Sci 2009;39:3–16.

10. Iribarren C, Jacobs DR Jr, Sidney S, Claxton AJ, Feingold KR. Cohort study of serum total cholesterol and in-hospital incidence of infectious diseases. Epidemiol Infect. 1998 Oct;121(2):335-47.

11. Ravnskov U, McCully KS. Infections may be causal in the pathogenesis of atherosclerosis. Am J Med Sci 2012;344:391–4.

Towards Revolutionary Understanding of Cellular Pathways in Health and Disease: Homocysteine Metabolism, Mitochondrial Dysfunction and the SAHACT Trial

Abdullah A. Alabdulgader, MD, DCH, MRCP, FRCP,
Kilmer S. Mccully, MD, Paul J. Rosch, MA, MD, FACP

Reviewing annual world health organization statistics on mortality and morbidity in the last few decades reveals an astonishing persistence of heart disease as the number one killer in all world nations and races. The substantial scientific advances in the last five decades contradict this disappointing fact. This means with no time for hesitation or comprehensive thinking, that the road map is wrong. Medical protocols and guidelines have improved longevity, but also increased the incidence of chronic diseases, and created new psychophysiological problems. Much of this is due to the influence of powerful pharmaceutical companies.

The historical background of the hypothesis of a causal relationship between the level of serum cholesterol and the development of atherosclerosis began with Rudolf Virchow's (1821-1902) description in 1856 of the atherosclerotic plaque with its cholesterol deposits. Nikolai Anitschkov's (1885–1964) experiments with rabbits in St Petersburg first demonstrated what was thought to be the role of cholesterol in the development of atherosclerosis. He fed rabbits cholesterol from egg yolks and found that they developed atherosclerotic plaques containing cholesterol. When he tried with other animals that were carnivores, it was not possible to reproduce the results. They didn't get atherosclerosis. In 1915 Anitschkov moved to Freiburg to work under Dr Aschoff, who at that time was considered the most accomplished of all German pathologists. This provided indirect support to his atherosclerosis theory.

A century has passed since the word "atherosclerosis" was introduced. It seems timely to revisit the early work of Anitschkov and his colleagues and to review their contribution to the total sum of our present understanding of one of the most dreadful human diseases. As reviewed by Kilmer McCully, Lewis Harry Newburgh (1898-1956) investigated the pioneering studies of cholesterol feeding to rabbits by Anitschkov during the period from 1915-1925. Newburgh and his team repeated the experiments of M. A. Ignatowsky (1880-1935), the investigator who first fed meat, milk and eggs to rabbits to produce arteriosclerotic plaques. Although Anitschkov attributed Ignatowsky's results to the cholesterol of the experimental diet, Newburgh's studies showed that removal of all fats and cholesterol from the experimental diet by extraction by organic solvents produced a protein powder that induced the same arteriosclerotic plaques observed by Ignatowsky. Newburgh's team injected pure amino acids intravenously in dogs and rabbits to determine which amino acid of the protein powder produced experimental arteriosclerotic plaques. No arterial plaques were demonstrated, but the animals developed chronic nephritis and albuminuria after injection of cysteine, tyrosine or tryptophan, confirming Ignatowsky's observations of nephritis in rabbits consuming a diet of meat, milk and eggs. Newburgh and his team failed to produce arterial plaques in his experiment, because the chemical structure of methionine and its presence in proteins were not determined until 1928. Moreover, the methionine derivative, homocysteine, was not discovered until 1932 by L. H. Butz and Vincent DuVigneaud (1901-1978) by demethylation of methionine by sulfuric acid. If Newburgh had been able to use methionine and homocysteine in his experiments in 1925, he undoubtedly would have discovered their ability to produce experimental arteriosclerotic plaques.

In 1953, Ancel Keys (1904-2004) reported that the dietary intake of fat was significantly correlated to the serum cholesterol level and the incidence of cardiovascular death in six countries. It appeared very convincing, but the problem was that 6 countries were selected from 22 that were available. There was no correlation when all the countries were included, and had he selected six others; he would have come to the opposite conclusion. The study was obviously falsified.

Another striking challenge of the cholesterol etiology of atherosclerosis came from studies of familial hypercholesterolemic population. Harlan *et al.*, in 1966, and later Mundal *et al.*, in 2014, reported that individuals with two to three times the normal level of LDL, have an overall normal rate of survival into their sixth, seventh, and even eighth decades of life. Indeed, Mundal *et al.* showed that individuals with FH from 70-79 years of age have a significantly lower rate of death than non-FH individuals with normal cholesterols. An elevated level of LDL does not cause coronary heart disease (CHD) or premature death. David Diamond and colleagues, who made an extensive review of FH literature, clearly pointed out the necessity of screening coagulation markers in those individuals, based on well-established evidence that a subset of FH individuals exhibit abnormal markers related to hypercoagulation. Given their higher risk of developing CHD, these FH individuals should be prioritized for interventions to optimize treatment that targets coagulopathy.

It became very clear that the true road map to fight against the number one world killer needed revolutionary thinking. A landmark publication in the field was published in 1969 by Kilmer McCully, who is often called the father of homocysteine theory in medicine, describing a new pathological mechanism leading to atherosclerosis called "Protein Intoxication due to high homocysteine in the blood". Homocysteine was named as an amino acid containing one extra carbon atom, in comparison with the similar chemical structure of cysteine, the amino acid which had previously first isolated from urinary bladder stones. Around the same time an eight-year-old boy of Irish-American ancestry admitted to Massachusetts General Hospital was evaluated for four days for headache, vomiting and drowsiness with signs of poor mental development in addition to dislocation of lenses in both eyes. Severe deterioration in the boy's condition with signs of stroke and weakness with abnormal reflexes on the left side were also reported. Furthermore, although there were no signs of infection, there was a rise in blood pressure and temperature; the boy succumbed to the illness within few days. The cause of death was reported as arteriosclerosis of the carotid artery with cerebral infarct; published as case 19,471 in the *New England Journal of Medicine* in 1933. It was found later that homocysteine is a sulphur containing amino acid derived from the essential amino acid methionine, present in large amounts in protein from animal sources like meat, eggs and milk. If there are adequate levels of vitamins B6, B12 and folic acid in the body, the homocysteine is broken down into harmless waste products or protein building blocks. But if there's a deficiency of those vitamins, the homocysteine begins its ravages on the blood vessels.

In retrospect, it seems clear that McCully was a man ahead of his time when everything focused on cholesterol. *"Kilmer McCully's hypothesis seemed to challenge the cholesterol-heart hypothesis, which was riding high,"* says Irwin Rosenberg, director of the U.S.D.A. Human Nutrition Research Center on Aging at Tufts University. His glorious discovery started when he became intrigued by two different cases of children with homocystinuria, a rare genetic disease in which the levels of homocysteine in the blood are unnaturally high. In both cases, the cause of death was severe arteriosclerosis, a narrowing and loss of elasticity in arteries that is normally seen only in the elderly. By re-examining the autopsy tissues of both children and drawing on previous animal research, McCully emerged with two linked and provocative suggestions: perhaps homocysteine directly damages the cells and tissues of the arteries, in much the way that cholesterol is thought to do, and perhaps that damage occurs not just in these rare genetic cases, but in the population at large, in anyone with an elevated homocysteine. He soon expanded his theory to include a probable cause of elevated levels of homocysteine: a deficiency of vitamins B6, B12 and folic acid. When these vitamins were administered to animals with high homocysteine levels, those levels plummeted, often within hours. Once McCully started extrapolating from his cellular-tissue and animal studies to the human situation, and said, *"it all began to fit together."* It is very clear now that high homocysteine is a pathological cause involved in a large spectrum of degenerative disorders. Numerous studies have demonstrated an association of high homocysteine with vascular disease, cancer and several age-related pathologies and neurodegenerative diseases, including Alzheimer's disease, Parkinson's disease, and dementia. Diabetes, Down syndrome, and megaloblastic anemia have also been linked to high levels of homocysteine. Additionally, there are studies showing an association between high homocysteine and osteoporosis, eye lens dislocation, end stage renal disease, insulin resistance, aneurysms, hypothyroidism, gastrointestinal and many other disorders.

The role of high homocysteine level in vascular injury and endothelial dysfunction is now clearer and has been attributed to impaired bioavailability of nitric oxide [NO]. One likely mechanism for reduced bioavailability of NO is mediated by asymmetric dimethylarginine (ADMA). This endogenous inhibitor of endothelial nitric oxide synthase (eNOS) competes with the natural substrate, L-arginine thus limiting the formation of NO. Elevated plasma levels of ADMA have been associated with hyperhomocysteinemia and endothelial dysfunction in both animals and humans. Apart from inhibiting the production of NO, ADMA may also promote the "uncoupling" of eNOS, thereby increasing the production of superoxide and other reactive oxygen species which in turn may further decrease NO bioavailability.

Recent advances have proven that there is a close link between hyperhomocystinuria and cancer. First, higher levels of plasma homocysteine have been observed in cancer patients, and venous thromboembolism (VTE) is the second most common cause of death in cancer patients. Second, several polymorphisms in the enzymes involved in the homocysteine detoxification pathways (the trans-sulfuration and remethylation) have close clinical ties to several types of cancer. Third, folate, which is pivotal for cell proliferation, has an inverse relation with homocysteine. Fourth, homocysteine has also been proposed as a potential tumor biomarker for a variety of cancers.

The hyperhomocysteinemia of aging and dementia is attributed to decreased synthesis of adenosyl methionine by thioretinaco ozonide and ATP, causing decreased allosteric activation of cystathionine synthase and decreased allosteric inhibition of methylenetetrahydrofolate reductase and resulting in dysregulation of methionine metabolism.

Mitochondria are the primary energy-producing organelles within human cells. Progressive mitochondrial dysfunction occurs in aging because of loss of the thioretinaco ozonide oxygen ATP complex from mitochondrial membranes by opening of the mitochondrial permeability transition pore (mPTP). Melatonin, a neuro-hormone, and cycloastragenol, a telomerase activator, both prevent mitochondrial dysfunction by inhibition of mPTP pore opening. The carcinogenic effects of radiofrequency radiation and mycotoxins are attributed to loss of thioretinaco ozonide from opening of the mPTP and decomposition of the active site of oxidative phosphorylation. The anti-aging effects of retinoids, the decreased concentration of cerebral cobalamin coenzymes in aging, and the diminished concentration of NAD+ from sirtuin activation, as observed in aging, all support the concept of loss of the thioretinaco ozonide oxygen ATP active site from mitochondria as the cause of decreased oxidative phosphorylation and mitochondrial dysfunction in aging.

In neurons, mitochondria are required for oxidative phosphorylation, intracellular calcium homeostasis, and regulation of cellular pH. Dysfunction of these organelles leads to cellular apoptosis through mechanisms such as intracellular reactive oxygen species generation and induction of the intrinsic apoptotic pathway. Mitochondrial dysfunction is implicated in the pathogenesis of many neurodegenerative disorders, including glaucoma, Alzheimer's disease, and Parkinson's disease. Interestingly, these diseases have been associated with elevated levels of plasma homocysteine. Homocysteine is thought to perturb the balance of mitochondrial fusion and fission in vivo. In retinal ganglion cells, this result in excessive mitochondrial fission and cellular apoptosis. Homocysteine appears to exert its actions by altering mitochondrial gene expression, function and structure.

Another recent molecular correlation was established between increased homocysteine levels in the blood and pulmonary embolism (PE). A Group of researchers examined the effects of homocysteine on PE pathogenesis and the molecular mechanisms underlying these effects. The results of the investigation demonstrated that 1 millimole of homocysteine significantly decreased cyclooxygenase (COX) activity and downregulated the expression of COX 17 in human umbilical vein endothelial cells. Decreased COX activity levels may lead to the elevation of intracellular reactive oxygen species (ROS) levels, further inducing apoptosis. It was seen that 1 millimole of homocysteine significantly increased the intracellular hydrogen peroxide (H2O2) level and the apoptosis rate in endothelial cells.

Homocysteine acts synergistically with H_2O_2 to exert some of its noxious effects and may modulate the cytotoxic effects of tumor necrosis factor (TNF). Cytokines such as TNF alpha may exert their cytotoxic effects by opening the permeability transition pore on the mitochondrial membrane thus uncoupling oxidative phosphorylation by dissipating the protonmotive force upon which ATP resynthesis depends. The beneficial effects of folic acid supplements in patients whose homocysteine levels are elevated can, therefore, be expected to be limited in those patients who have other causes of an impairment of oxidative phosphorylation.

In the quinquagenarian celebration of what Kilmer McCully described as" protein Intoxication" and the accumulated explosive scientific evidence – since then – of the causal relationship of abnormal homocysteine blood levels and the widespread human pathologies combined with the unequivocal cellular pathways derangements associated with hyperhomocysteinemia, we are facing historical obligations and responsibilities. This emerging level of evidence contradicts the faulty, scrawny and meager scientific evidence for the cholesterol theory of atherosclerosis. It is coming after a decade of my first meeting with Kilmer McCully in the Third King of Organs International Conference for Advanced Cardiac Sciences 2010. The King of Organs series of conferences was founded and chaired by us in the years 2006, 2008, 2010, 2012 and 2019. Turning points in the journey of human sciences emerged from King of Organ Conferences. One of those turning points was **The Saudi Arabian Homocysteine Atherosclerosis and Cancer Clinical Trial (SAHACT)**. The father of homocysteine theory in modern medicine, Kilmer McCully is again the father of SAHACT. Abdullah Alabdulgader is the principal Investigator of SAHACT. Paul Rosch is our honorary consultant and teacher in the field. Considering his magnificent input to the homocysteine science we are honored to add him as co-author of this chapter.

The objective of SAHACT is to utilize a nutritional-metabolic multicenter clinical interventional trial to demonstrate how therapeutic strategies for controlling homocysteine metabolism are effective in prevention and treatment of degenerative diseases associated with aging. New understanding of the importance of retinol (vitamin A), ascorbate (vitamin C), and homocysteine thiolactone in the biosynthesis of thioretinamide and thioretinaco by cystathionine synthase suggests a promising method for control of abnormal homocysteine metabolism in human subjects with arteriosclerosis and cancer.

The recent advances and knowledge of mitochondrial functions and dysfunctions were incorporated intelligently in SAHACT. The efficacy of pancreatic enzyme therapy of cancer is interpreted as a promising method for promoting catabolism of macromolecules, specifically proteins, nucleic acids, and glycosaminoglycans that contain excess homocysteine groups resulting from abnormal accumulation of homocysteine thiolactone in aging, atherogenesis and carcinogenesis.

Dietary deficiencies of nitriloside (vitamin B17), folate (vitamin B9), pyridoxal (vitamin B6), and cobalamin (vitamin B12) contribute to abnormal homocysteine metabolism in degenerative diseases. Dietary deficiency of proteins containing sulfur amino acids down-regulates cystathionine synthase, causing abnormal homocysteine metabolism and increased risk of cardiovascular disease. Infections by a variety of micro-organisms promote abnormal homocysteine metabolism in atherogenesis and carcinogenesis, leading to creation of vulnerable plaques of arteries and dysplastic transformation of susceptible cells of various organs.

The protocol of the SAHACT trial consists of retinol, thioretinamide, and cobalamin as precursors of thioretinaco, combined with pancreatic enzyme extracts, nutritional modification to eliminate processed foods and to enhance dietary consumption of nitrilosides and other vitamins, and combined with vitamin supplements, essential amino acids, beneficial dietary fats, beneficial dietary protein, and antibiotics to combat chronic infections. Groups of subjects with vascular disease will be randomized into treatment with the nutritional-metabolic protocol versus usual therapy, and outcome will be followed for prevention of adverse vascular events, including acute coronary syndrome, stroke and amputation. Groups of subjects with recurrent prostate cancer or breast cancer will be randomized into treatment with the nutritional-metabolic protocol versus usual therapy, and outcome will be followed for prevention of mortality and complications of cancer.

The SAHACT trial is designed to demonstrate the efficacy of a novel nutritional-metabolic approach to prevention and therapy of the important degenerative diseases of aging, arteriosclerosis and cancer. This approach will be compared with current methods of therapy for these diseases in a randomized, prospective, multicenter clinical interventional trial. The advantage of this novel approach is the non-toxic nature of the methods, utilizing vitamins, vitamin derivatives, amino acids, beneficial fats and proteins, essential amino acids, and antibiotics to achieve prevention and therapy. The design of the trial permits direct comparison of outcomes of the SAHACT protocols with the outcomes of conventional therapy with cholesterol-lowering drugs and other measures for prevention of vascular disease, and outcomes of chemotherapy, hormone therapy, radiation therapy and ·

surgery for malignant disease. Successful completion of the SAHACT trial will for the first time allow consideration of this innovative protocol for prevention and treatment of degenerative diseases of aging in susceptible populations in humankind worldwide.

The nutritional-metabolic concept of SAHCT is based on the understanding of the function of thioretinamide, thioretinaco, and thioretinaco ozonide in the metabolic origin of degenerative diseases, including arteriosclerosis, stroke, acute coronary syndrome, cancer, dementia and other neurodegenerative diseases, autoimmune diseases such as ulcerative colitis, lupus erythematosus, thyroiditis, rheumatoid arthritis and pernicious anaemia, osteoporosis and fracture, venous thrombosis and embolism, retinal vein thrombosis, macular degeneration, hypothyroidism, accelerated aging, renal failure and uremia, diabetes mellitus, metabolic syndrome, severe psoriasis, organ transplantation with therapeutic immune suppression, protein energy malnutrition, familial or spontaneous amyloidosis, dietary deficiencies of folate, pyridoxal, and cobalamin, complications of pregnancy such as placenta previa and pre-eclampsia, and congenital birth defects including neural tube defects, cleft palate, and congenital heart disease. In each of these degenerative diseases and conditions, abnormal homocysteine metabolism has been demonstrated by an increased level of homocysteine bound to plasma proteins by disulphide bonds.

SAHACT is adopting intelligent scientific directions incorporating the human cellular pathways in health and disease to combat the pathological process of degenerative disorders, most importantly atherosclerosis and cancer. The role of mitochondrial dysfunction in aging and degenerative diseases is key to our understanding of the SAHACT protocol.

Elucidation of trophoblastic origin of malignant cells was utilized in SAHACT intelligently. The trophoblastic origin of malignant cells, as described by the embryologist John Beard, was incorporated in the therapeutic goals of SAHACT. This is based on the premise that trophoblastic cells of the embryo, which invade the uterine endometrium and myometrium during implantation of the fertilized embryo, are related to the asexual cycle of cellular organisms and are converted to placental cytotrophoblastic and syncytiotrophoblastic cells by the action of enzymes produced by the pancreas of the developing fetus. Based on the concept that trophoblastic cells, which are distributed within developing tissues of the fetus, are similar in their cellular behavior to malignant cells, Beard introduced the enzyme therapy of cancer. This treatment consists of injecting enzymes and pro-enzymes extracted from porcine pancreas into patients with various forms of primary or metastatic cancer. The trophoblastic theory of the origin of cancer is based on the assumption that adult stem cells are related to the trophoblastic cells which migrate from the yolk sac of the developing embryo into somatic tissues, as described by Beard.

Human fetal and malignant cells produce small quantities of chorionic gonadotrophin. This hormone is produced in large quantities by the highly malignant tumor of placenta, choriocarcinoma. These observations provide additional evidence for the trophoblastic origin of malignant cells. Although the origin of adult stem cells in normal human tissues is currently not well understood, the sensitivity of trophoblastic cells to oncolysis by pancreatic enzymes and pro-enzymes forms the theoretical basis for this therapeutic approach. This sensitivity is related to the accumulation of homocysteinylated enzymes, plasma proteins, and cellular proteins, ribonucleic acid, deoxyribonucleic acid, and glycosaminoglycans by reaction with excess homocysteine thiolactone that accumulates during aging, atherogenesis, carcinogenesis, and autoimmune diseases. Pancreatic extracts contain active trypsin, chymotrypsin, elastase, amylase, lipase, ribonuclease, and deoxyribonuclease, as well as proenzyme precursors of these digestive enzymes. These enzymes are capable of hydrolyzing the homocysteinated proteins, nucleic acids and glycosaminoglycans that accumulate in malignant tissues and in the tissues of aging persons.

The discovery of thioretinamide, thioretinaco and thioretinaco ozonide and its antineoplastic properties was incorporated in the SAHACT protocol. Homocysteine thiolactone reacts with retinoic acid to form N-homocysteine thiolactonyl retinamide (NHTR), known as thioretinamide, in organic synthesis. Thioretinamide reacts with cobalamin to form N-homocysteine thiolactonyl retinamido cobalamin ((NHTR)2Cbl), known as thioretinaco. Both thioretinamide and thioretinaco have anti-carcinogenic and anti-neoplastic activities in mice treated with a carcinogen and in mice with transplanted neoplasms.

The accumulated knowledge on ascorbate, homocysteine thiolactone oxidation, and growth hormone properties as anticancer factors was added to strengthen the SAHACT protocol. In the 1930s, ascorbic acid was found to influence the growth of cancer in animals, mainly acting to extend longevity. Moreover, the amount of ascorbic acid in the tissues of animals with cancer is decreased, further suggesting the possibility of a therapeutic action in cancer patients. Otto Warburg discovered the role of cytochrome enzymes in cellular respiration. He later demonstrated that cancer cells and embryonic cells have a characteristic mode of cellular respiration known as aerobic glycolysis in which glucose is converted to lactic acid instead of conversion to carbon dioxide, as seen in normal cells. Ascorbic acid inhibits cellular respiration and glycolysis of cancer cells. Early and controversial studies claimed that massive doses of ascorbic acid cause regression of some advanced human cancers and extended the life span of patients with terminal malignancies, compared with controls. Subsequent controlled studies showed that massive doses of ascorbic acid have minor effects on side effects of chemotherapy and radiation and produce a slight increase in survival times of cancer patients.

The advances in understanding the pathways of glycolysis, nitrilosides, and hydrogen sulfide role in malignant cells is integral to the SAHACT protocol.

In the early 20th century Warburg discovered that embryonic tissues and malignant cells are unable to utilize oxygen for cellular metabolism but instead metabolize glucose to lactate as a source of cellular energy. In other studies, Warburg showed that carcinogenic chemicals decrease normal cellular respiration by irreversible inhibition of oxygenases and by irreversible inhibition of transport of electrons by cytochrome enzyme systems. These findings are supported by the demonstration of deficient succinic dehydrogenase and cytochrome oxidase activities within malignant tissues. Taken together these early observations can be interpreted as examples of the clonal selection of malignant cells from trophoblastic stem cells that are deficient in the heme oxidase activity of cystathionine synthase. The resulting failure of oxidation of retinol to retinoic acid and failure of reaction of retinoic acid with homocysteine thiolactone to produce thioretinamide by these malignant cells will lead to deficient formation of thioretinaco and failure of oxidative phosphorylation, catalyzed by thioretinaco ozonide. The failure of oxidative phosphorylation by malignant cell clones that are deficient in the heme oxygenase function of cystathionine synthase, resulting from decreased production of thioretinaco ozonide from cobalamin and thioretinamide, will lead to an embryonic form of metabolism in which ATP synthesis is dependent upon production of lactate from glucose, otherwise known as aerobic glycolysis.

Nitrilosides are substances containing nitrile groups produced by plants. The most important plant nitriloside is amygdalin (mandelonitrile β-diglucoside), and other nitrilosides are dhurrin (hydroxymandelonitrile β-glucoside), lotaustralin (methylethyl-ketone-cyanohydrin β-glucoside), and linamarin (acetone-cyanohydrin β-glucoside). Malignant cells contain glucosidase, the enzyme that metabolizes amygdalin and other nitrilosides to cyanide. Normal cells contain rhodanese, a sulfotransferase enzyme that catalyzes thiocyanate synthesis from cyanide and hydrogen sulfide. Malignant cells contain insufficient rhodanese to prevent accumulation of cyanide. Therefore, the prevention and control of growth of malignant cells and tissues by dietary nitrilosides are attributable to the consequent accumulation of cyanide within malignant cells. The reaction of cyanide with the cobalt atom of thioretinaco inactivates thioretinaco ozonide, thereby preventing oxidative phosphorylation.

This system of chemical surveillance against the growth of trophoblastic malignant cell clones is promoted by dietary or supplemental consumption of amygdalin and other plant nitrilosides. Hydrogen sulphide is generated from homocysteine by cystathionine synthase and cystathionase, and low levels of hydrogen sulphide decrease oxidative stress and ameliorate pathological conditions such as ischemia-reperfusion injury, hypertension, and renal failure. Hydrogen sulphide is a key gasotransmitter in sensing oxygen availability in tissues. The reducing properties of hydrogen sulphide are responsible for scavenging the reactive oxygen species production induced by increased blood levels of homocysteine, inhibiting myocardial injury. Increased production of hydrogen sulphide from homocysteine, metabolized from homocysteinylated proteins, nucleic acids, and glycosaminoglycans of apoptotic cells by pancreatic enzymes will promote catabolism of homocysteine and conversion of the sulfur atom of homocysteine to thiocyanate by reaction of hydrogen sulphide with the cyanide generated from dietary nitrilosides.

The role of homocysteine, thioretinamide, and thioretinaco in degenerative diseases is the cornerstone of the SAHACT scientific protocol

108

The etiology of many of these degenerative diseases and conditions is incompletely understood. However, many of these chronic degenerative diseases are strongly correlated with the aging process. The importance of deficiencies of thioretinaco ozonide in cells of aging tissues is related to accumulation of homocysteine thiolactone and homocysteinylation of macromolecules. Regardless of etiology, however, elevation of plasma homocysteine levels and homocysteinylation of macromolecules in chronic degenerative diseases are susceptible to therapeutic intervention by preservation of cellular oxidative metabolism through increased production of thioretinaco ozonide and by enhanced catabolism of homocysteine produced by enzymatic degradation of homocysteinylated macromolecules. Moreover, preservation of cellular thioretinaco ozonide by membranergic proteins and by the liposomal complex of ATP and oxygen with thioretinaco prolongs survival and counteracts the aging process.

The role of infectious organisms in the pathogenesis of arteriosclerotic plaques was considered carefully in the SAHACT protocol.

Vulnerable plaques of arteries in atherosclerosis originate from obstruction of *vasa vasorum* of arterial wall by aggregates formed from lipoproteins complexed with microbial remnants, homocysteinylated lipoproteins, and lipoprotein autoantibodies in areas of high tissue pressure, causing ischemia, degeneration of arterial wall cells and rupture into arterial intima to form a micro-abscess. The evidence that human arteriosclerotic plaques contain ozone supports the theoretical role of ozone in activation of thioretinaco to form thioretinaco ozonide as the active site for oxidative phosphorylation.

As a matter of fact, SAHACT represents a promising innovative approach to control degenerative diseases of aging that has never been studied in human trials. The work of Kilmer McCully over the past five decades has focused on understanding the underlying abnormalities of homocysteine metabolism in degenerative diseases by studies of pathological anatomy of arteries in human and experimental hyperhomocysteinemia, by studies of homocysteine metabolism in cell cultures, in physiological animal experiments, and by studies of experimental atherogenesis and carcinogenesis in animal models. SAHACT trial is testing for the first time this approach in human disease. No similar trial has been proposed by any other investigator or research team to our knowledge. The clarity of the cellular pathways of homocysteine metabolism in health and disease and the ability of the researchers in the last half decade to establish unequivocally the pathogenic role of what was described in 1969 as "Protein Intoxication" are compulsive historical messages to the international community to find pathways that will cure or at least ameliorate the devastating effects of degenerative diseases. This is in contrast to the fallacious cholesterol hypothesis, which has no proven scientific support of a causal role. It is merely an epidemiological created correlation contaminated by cherry picking, selective data management, skewed with statistical deception. It is no surprise that efforts to treat this false assumption have resulted in massive epidemics of cardiac and non-cardiovascular diseases.

SAHACT is creating the first true footstep to introduce intelligent alternative therapeutic approaches based on nature and natural products, to replace the highly toxic and poisonous chemicals and radiation therapies to treat degenerative diseases.

Abdullah A. Alabdulgader* MD, DCH, MRCP, FRCP, Kilmer S. McCully**, MD, Paul J. Rosch***, MA, MD, FACP

* Senior Scientist, Interventional Congenital Cardiologist, Electrophysiologist, cryo and robotic ablation specialist and electrical devices implanter. Principal Investigator of SAHACT, Prince Sultan Cardiac Center, Alhasa, Saudi Arabia

** Father of Homocysteine in modern medicine. Pathology and Laboratory Medicine Service, Boston Veterans Affairs Medical Center, and Department of Pathology, Harvard Medical School, Boston, MA, USA

*** Clinical Professor of Medicine and Psychiatry, New York Medical College, Valhalla, NY, USA
Chairman of the Board, The American Institute of Stress, Weatherford, TX, USA
Honorary Vice President, International Society of Stress Management. London, UK

Editor's Note

From Abdullah A. Alabdulgader.
The protocol and science for SAHACT (Saudi Arabian Homocysteine Atherosclerosis and Cancer Trial), which was devised by Dr Kilmer McCully, was approved with a very high rating (13.5/15) by the Research Competitiveness Science and Policy Program Committee of the American Association for the Advancement of Science in July 2011. It received IRB approval from KACST (King Abdulaziz City of Science and Technology-Regional IRB of Prince Sultan Cardiac Center) in October 2018. Abdullah Alabdulgader was assigned principal investigator as Congress President (where SAHACT was first proposed and submitted), since a Saudi citizen is required to supervise the scientific and administrative protocols of the trial in hospitals. Dr McCully was assigned as Senior Consultant and Dr Paul Rosch as Honorary Consultant. This chapter is based on a presentation by Dr Alabdulgader at the March 2019 Fifth International Congress for Advanced Cardiac Sciences (King of Organs 2019) and includes additional comments from Drs. McCully and Rosch.

Suggested reading:

1. McCully KS. Hyperhomocysteinemia and arteriosclerosis: historical perspectives. Clinical Chemistry and Laboratory Medicine 2005;43:980-986.

2. Beard J. *The Enzymatic Treatment of Cancer and its Scientific Basis* Chatto & Windus, London, 1911, republished by New Spring Press, New York, 2010 with a foreword by Nicholas Gonzalez.

3. Novak JF, Trynka F. Proenzyme therapy of cancer. Anticancer Res 2005;25:1157-1178.

4. Gonzalez N, Isaacs L. *The Trophoblast and the Origins of Cancer.* New Spring Press, New York, 2009.

5. McCully KS. Vascular pathology of homocysteinemia: implications for the pathogenesis of arteriosclerosis. Am J Pathol 1969;56:111-128.

6. Kilmer S. McCully: Homocysteine Thiolactone Metabolism in Malignant Cells. CANCER RESEARCH 36, 3198-3202, September 1976.

7. Ganapathy PS, Perry RL, Tawfik A, *et al.* Homocysteine-mediated modulation of mitochondrial dynamics in retinal ganglion cells. *Invest Ophthalmol Vis Sci.* 2011;52(8):5551–5558. Published 2011 Jul 25. doi:10.1167/iovs.11-7256

8. Yang, F., Qi, X., Gao, Z., Yang, X., Zheng, X., Duan, C., Zheng, J. "Homocysteine injures vascular endothelial cells by inhibiting mitochondrial activity". Experimental and Therapeutic Medicine 12.4 (2016): 2247-2252.

9. McCully KS. Review: Chemical Pathology of Homocysteine VI. Aging, Cellular Senescence, and Mitochondrial Dysfunction. Ann Clin Lab Sci. 2018 Sep;48(5):677-687.

10. McCully KS. The active site of oxidative phosphorylation and the origin of hyperhomocysteinemia in aging and dementia. Ann Clin Lab Sci. 2015 Spring;45(2):222-5.

11. Ping Zhang, Zhen Huang, Yongkun Gui, Bin Zhu, Haiqing Yan, Xiaolu Niu, Xuejing Yue, Tong Li, Yuming Xu. Correlation between levels of serum homocystein, high sensitivity C-reactive protein and subtypes of large artery atherosclerosis ischemic stroke. Life Sci J 2013;10(1):3145-3149] (ISSN:1097-8135).http://www.lifesciencesite.com.

12. McCully KS. Homocysteine Metabolism, Atherosclerosis, and Diseases of Aging. Compr Physiol. 2015 Dec 15;6(1):471-505. doi: 10.1002/cphy.c150021.

13. McCully KS. Homocysteine, Infections, Polyamines, Oxidative Metabolism, and the Pathogenesis of Dementia and Atherosclerosis. J Alzheimers Dis. 2016 Oct 18;54(4):1283-1290.

14. McCully KS. Hyperhomocysteinemia, Suppressed Immunity, and Altered Oxidative Metabolism Caused by Pathogenic Microbes in Atherosclerosis and Dementia. Front Aging Neurosci. 2017 Oct 6;9:324. doi: 10.3389/fnagi.2017.00324. eCollection 2017.

15. McCully KS. Loss of the Thioretinaco Ozonide Oxygen Adenosine Triphosphate Complex from Mitochondria Produces Mitochondrial Dysfunction and Carcinogenesis. Ann Clin Lab Sci. 2018 May;48(3):386-393.

Saturated Fat and Coronary Heart Disease in Europe

Zoë Harcombe, PhD

In March 2015, I decided to repeat an exercise that Dr Malcolm Kendrick had done for his 2008 book "The Great Cholesterol Con."[1] In this book, Dr Kendrick reviewed the top and bottom seven countries for saturated fat intake in Europe and the countries with the highest and lowest levels of heart deaths. He found that the top seven countries for saturated fat intake all had lower rates of heart disease than the bottom seven countries for saturated fat intake. Why Seven Countries? To mirror the famous Keys' Seven Countries Study.[2]

Dr Kendrick used the MONICA data from c. 1998. I repeated the exercise using the 2008 data.[3] The data were available for Europe for men and women and for Coronary Heart Disease (CHD).[4]

First, I did a scatter plot and trend line for the 44 countries in Europe for which data were available. As you can see from the charts, the association is inverse – the higher the saturated fat intake, the lower the CHD death rate for males...

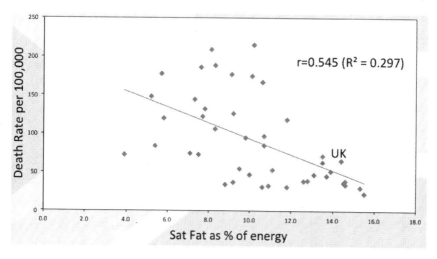

FIGURE 1 **European data for CHD deaths and sat fat (males)**

113

and for females...

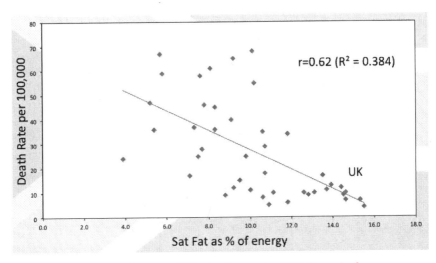

FIGURE 2 European data for CHD deaths and sat fat (females)

The correlation for males (r) is 0.55 and it is even stronger (0.62) for females.

The top and bottom seven

Then I repeated Kendrick's Seven Countries study:

- The seven countries with the *lowest* saturated fat intake were Bosnia & Herzegovinia; Georgia; Tajikstan; Azerbaijan; Moldova; Croatia; Armenia.

- Their saturated fat intake ranged from 3.9-7.3%. The average was 5.8% – all well below the recommended 10% saturated fat limit set by dietary guidelines.

- The seven countries with the *highest* saturated fat intake were France; Switzerland; Netherlands; Iceland; Belgium; Finland; Austria (France is the single country with the highest saturated fat intake in Europe and the lowest rate of CHD deaths).

- Their saturated fat intake ranged from 13.9-15.5%. The average was 14.7% – all well above the recommended 10% saturated fat limit set by dietary guidelines.

- The 7 countries with the *lowest* saturated fat intake had the following death rates:

  ○ Male deaths per 100,000 ranged from 73-178, with an average death rate of 117.

  ○ Female deaths per 100,000 ranged from 17-67, with an average death rate of 41.

- The 7 countries with the highest saturated fat intake had the following death rates:

  ○ Male deaths per 100,000 ranged from 22-65, with an average death rate of 39.

  ○ Female deaths per 100,000 ranged from 4-13, with an average death rate of 9.

Lowest SFA intake (3.9-7.3%)	Highest SFA intake (13.9-15.5%)
Bosnia & Herzegovinia	France
Georgia	Switzerland
Tajikstan	Netherlands
Azerbaijan	Iceland
Moldova	Belgium
Croatia	Finland
Armenia	Austria
Average SFA intake 5.8%	*Average SFA intake 14.7%*
Men: 117 CHD deaths per 100,000	*Men: 39 CHD deaths per 100,000*
Women: 41 per 100,000	*Women: 9 per 100,000*

Death rates for men were 3 times higher in the lowest saturated fat intake countries than the highest.

Death rates for women were 4.5 times higher in the lowest saturated fat intake countries than the highest.

As Kendrick found from the 1998 data – every single country in the top seven saturated fat intake countries had a lower death rate than every single country in the bottom seven saturated fat intake countries. This held for men and women. It held again with the data from 10 years on.

Zoë Harcombe, PhD

Independent Researcher
www.zoeharcombe.com

References

1. http://www.zoeharcombe.com/2015/03/saturated-fat-chd-in-europe/

2. Keys *et al.*, "The Seven Countries Study: Volumes I-XX", Circulation, (April 1970).

3. Allender S, Scarborough P, Peto V, Rayner M. European Cardiovascular Disease Statistics: British Heart Foundation Health Promotion Research Group, 2008.

4. Allender S, Scarborough P, Peto V, Rayner M. European Cardiovascular Disease Statistics: British Heart Foundation Health Promotion Research Group, 2008.

Part Three

The Benefits of Cholesterol and
The Dangers of Statins

Why Cholesterol is our Best Friend

Uffe Ravnskov, MD PhD

Don't do this and don't do that
What are they trying to do? – Make a good boy of you
Do they know where it's at?
Don't criticize, they're old and wise
Do as they tell you to
Don't want the devil to
Come and put out your eyes

Roger Hodgson

For more than half a century high cholesterol has been considered as the main cause of atherosclerosis and cardiovascular disease, and that the most important way of prevention is to lower it as much as possible; the lower, the better. But is it true?

As the famous philosopher Karl Popper stated, a medical hypothesis cannot be proved, but it can be falsified. If it cannot be falsified, it is not a scientific hypothesis. If your hypothesis says that all swans are white, it has been falsified when you find a black one. The cholesterol hypothesis is indeed scientific, because it is possible to falsify it, and it has indeed been falsified again and again for many years but apparently very few scientists have realized that. Let me therefore tell you about the many falsifications. References to all of the studies mentioned are available in four studies which I have published in cooperation with 16 international experts. Links to some of these papers are available at the end of the chapter.

The first and strongest falsification was shown more than 80 years ago. If high cholesterol is the cause of atherosclerosis, there should be exposure-response; people with high cholesterol should of course become more atherosclerotic than people with low cholesterol; this is self-evident. But here is what the American researchers Landé and

Sperry found. They analysed the amount of cholesterol present in the aorta in more than one hundred dead people and compared it with the level of cholesterol in their blood. What they found was that those with low cholesterol had just as much cholesterol in their arteries as those with high cholesterol. But the few who remember Landé and Sperry claim that cholesterol values in dead people are not identical with those in living people.

However, their finding has been verified by at least a dozen research groups whose cholesterol was measured before they died. For instance, in a Canadian study, Paterson and his co-workers followed elderly people for several years and analysed their cholesterol several times during the observation period. When they died, they performed a similar analysis as did Landé and Sperry and with the same result. It is a simple fact that people with low cholesterol become just as atherosclerotic as people with high cholesterol.[1]

Some researchers have claimed that there is an association, but these studies have been performed on hospital patients, where the number with familial hypercholesterolemia (inherited high cholesterol) are much larger than in the general population. A few people with this abnormality are more atherosclerotic than normal people, but it is not due to their high cholesterol. This appears from many studies because when the data from those with familial hypercholesterolemia are separated from the data from people without this abnormality, the association between cholesterol and degree of atherosclerosis disappears in both groups.

There is not even an association between degree of calcification and serum cholesterol. In fact, in an American study, there was a weak *inverse* association; cholesterols of those with the lowest degree of calcification were a little higher than cholesterols of those with the highest degree of calcification. I sent a short letter to the editor of the journal where this study was published asking him why they haven't commented anything about this striking finding. He answered that *"because of space limitations we are able to publish only a few letters addressing controversial issues."*[1]

High cholesterol and high LDL-cholesterol are also considered as the most important risk factors for cardiovascular disease. Here many researchers refer to the Framingham study in which the authors found that cholesterols of those who died from a heart attack were

120

slightly higher than normal. However, in a 30-year follow-up of the participants in that study, the authors wrote that *"for each 1 mg/dl drop in cholesterol per year, there was an eleven percent increase in coronary and total mortality."*[1]

But in a review published by the American Heart Association and the National Heart, Lung, and Blood Institute three years later you can read the following: *"A one percent reduction in an individual's TC results in an approximate two percent reduction in CHD* (coronary Heart disease) *risk"*, and as support they referred to the 30-year follow-up study from Framingham, which had found the opposite![1]

In accordance with the findings of the 30-year report from Framingham, many studies have shown that high cholesterol is not a risk factor for heart disease, particularly among people who have reached the age where these diseases start to occur. On my home page[2] you can find more than 25 references to such studies.

Somebody might say that it is a high level of LDL-cholesterol that is important. But that is impossible because in a paper published in the *British Medical Journal*,[3] we showed that after the age of 60, those with the highest LDL-cholesterols lived the longest. This was the result of 19 studies including more than 68,000 elderly people. Our paper has been heavily criticised by many statin-advocates all over the world, but nobody has been able to point at any study with the opposite result.[3]

Furthermore, several studies have shown that on average, LDL-cholesterol is lower than normal in patients with acute myocardial infarction. In one of these studies the authors were concerned, and decided to lower cholesterol even more. At follow-up three years later, twice as many with the lowest LDL-cholesterol had died compared to those with the highest LDL-cholesterol.[1]

A relevant question is why many studies have shown that high cholesterol or high LDL-cholesterol is a risk factor among younger people. Most likely, stress is the explanation. On average, younger people are more stressed than elderly people and stress is able to raise cholesterol by 30-40% in the course of half an hour, and stress may also cause atherosclerosis by other mechanisms.[1]

But what about the trials, you may ask. Haven't our opponents demonstrated in more than 30 statin trials that lowering cholesterol is able to lower the risk of cardiovascular disease? Isn't it the strongest proof of the cholesterol hypothesis?

There are major problems with these trials, however. For example, none of them have succeeded with prolonging the life of women or healthy people of either sex. Furthermore, if high cholesterol was the cause of atherosclerosis and cardiovascular disease, the benefit should of course be higher the more it is lowered; e.g. there should be exposure-response. But exposure-response has only been calculated in three statin trials, and none of them showed this, and in more than a dozen angiographic trials where exposure-response was calculated, only one of them found exposure-response, and the only treatment in that trial was exercise.[1]

In a recent review by the American researcher Brian Ference and his co-workers they claimed there was exposure-response. Although they referred to 33 trials in the text, in the figure which they used as proof, they had included data from only 12 trials. In our recent review,[1] we have calculated exposure-response with data from all of the trials and found that there was no exposure-response. A relevant question is, if this way of deliberate misinformation is used because the European Atherosclerosis Society, which had organised the review, has been taken over by Big Pharma because with one exception, all of the 26 authors of the review were supported financially by the drug industry.

Many of the statin-reports are in conflict with the findings by independent researchers and they have therefore asked for the primary data, but this hasn't been allowed by the drug industry. In 2005 new international regulations were introduced according to which everyone has access to the primary data. Since then, no statin trial has succeeded in lowering mortality.[1]

After our publication in the *British Medical Journal*,[1] the statin advocates have obviously become desperate. Several large reviews have been published in which the cholesterol lies have been repeated again and again. I have already mentioned the review by Brian Ference and his co-workers. Another one is a 120-pages long repetition of the cholesterol guidelines by Scott Grundy and 23 co-authors. The surprising news is that none of them seems to have any financial conflicts. This appears from a large table filling more than two pages.

But beneath the table you can read the following in small letters:

The table does not necessarily reflect relationships with industry at the time of publication. A person is deemed to have a significant interest in a business if the interest represents ownership of ≥5% of the voting stock or share of the business *entity, or ownership of ≥$5,000 of the fair market value of the business entity; or if funds received by the person from the business entity exceed 5% of the person's gross income for the previous year.*

One of the commonest arguments in support of the statins is that cardiovascular mortality has decreased because of the introduction of these drugs. However, heart mortality had already started to decrease in the seventies, and there has not been any change in the mortality curve following the introduction of the statins in the early nineties. The cause of the decrease is most likely lesser smoking and better treatment of acute cardiovascular disease.

According to the statin trials, almost all of which are funded by drug companies, side effects are extremely rare – less than 0.1%. However, most of them have started with a run-in period where those who experienced side effects were excluded. But in the IDEAL trial they obviously forgot to do this. It was a trial in which a high statin dose was compared with a low statin dose. In that trial, almost 50% in each group suffered from serious side effects (Table 1).[1]

	High dose atorvastatin No. (%)	Usual dose simvastatin No. (%)
Any adverse effect	4204 (94.4)	4202 (94.4)
Any serious adverse event	2064 (46.6)	2108 (47.4)

TABLE 1 **Number of side effects in the IDEAL trial according to table 4 in the trial report**

This information wasn't mentioned either in the text or in the abstract; only in the Table, and if you retrieve the paper from the web, you will only get access to the Tables if you select the PDF version.

Here are some of the side effects, most of which have been reported by independent researchers: muscle pain, rhabdomyolysis, kidney failure, liver failure, diabetes, hearing loss, cataract, heart failure, cancer, memory loss, cognitive impairment, aggressive behaviour, depression, Parkinson, ALS, dementia and peripheral nerve damage. The large number of cerebral dysfunctions isn't unexpected because the highest concentration of cholesterol is located in the brain.[4]

123

The most serious side effect is probably cancer. Statin supporters usually claim that high cholesterol predispose to cancer. The question therefore is, why after only a few years of treatment, cancer occurred significantly more frequently in four of the first statin trials (Table 2).[1]

Statin trial	Age of the participants (years)	Type of cancer	Number of cancers Treatment group	Control group
CARE	21-75	Breast	12 (4.1%)	1 (0.05%)
4S+HPS	35-80	Skin	256 (2.5%)	208 (1,66%)
PROSPER	70-82	All	245 (11,81%)	199 (9,12%)

TABLE 2 **The number of new cancer cases in four statin trials, where the difference was statistically significant. The results from 4S and HPS are combined**

But what about familial hypercholesterolemia, you may ask. Doesn't the high heart mortality among people with this abnormality prove that high cholesterol causes atherosclerosis and cardiovascular disease?

Together with three colleagues I have examined the medical literature about familial hypercholesterolemia systematically for many years without finding any evidence that their risk of heart disease is due to their high cholesterol.[5] What we found was that, just as is the case in normal people, there is no association between degree of atherosclerosis and LDL-cholesterol, and in most studies, LDL-cholesterol of those who had suffered from coronary heart disease was not higher than LDL-cholesterol of those who did not suffer. Furthermore, people with familial hypercholesterolemia are said to die early from cardiovascular disease, although it has been shown that on average they live just as long as other people. For instance, here are the figures from Simon Broome's register group, who followed 2,234 individuals with familial hypercholesterolemia for 4.3 years prior to the introduction of statins, and compared their heart mortality rates with those in the general population.

Age (years)	Observed number of deaths	Expected number of deaths
20-39	6	0.06
40-59	8	1.54
60-74	1	2.28

TABLE 3 Number of deaths caused by coronary heart disease among 2,234 individuals with familial hypercholesterolemia and in the general population during 4.3 years observation time before the introduction of the statin drugs according to the Simon Broome Register group[5]

As you see, up to age 59, only fourteen among 1,884 individuals with familial hypercholesterolemia had died from heart disease during these years, and only one among the 358 individuals between age 60 and 74 years.

But why do younger people with familial hypercholesterolemia die earlier than normal people if it isn't due to their high cholesterol, you may ask. One of the reasons is that those who die early have also inherited high levels of various coagulation factors. Therefore, there are no reasons to lower their cholesterol. With one exception, no controlled randomised cholesterol-lowering trial including only people with familial hypercholesterolemia has been successful. The exception is a trial using apheresis, a technique where the blood is passed through an apparatus that separates out particular constituents, for instance cholesterol, but this technique also removes several coagulation factors as well.

Our conclusion is that the statements from the supporters of the cholesterol campaign and the drug companies are invalid. They are compromised by misleading statistics, by excluding unsuccessful trials, by minimizing the side effects of cholesterol lowering, and by ignoring hundreds of contradictory observations from independent investigators.

Hopefully, the world's health authorities will have the courage to stop the cholesterol campaign, because the crises in the health care system today in many countries may be caused by dietary misinformation and by the prescription of a drug with many serious side effects to millions and millions of healthy people all over the world.

Uffe Ravnskov, MD PhD

References

1. Ravnskov U, de Lorgeril M, Diamond DM *et al.* LDL-C does not cause cardiovascular disease: a comprehensive review of current literature. Expert Rev Clin Pharmacol. 2018;11:959-70. https://www.tandfonline.com/doi/pdf/10.1080/17512433.2018.1519391?needAccess=true

2. www.ravnskov.nu/2015/12/27/myth-9

3. Ravnskov U, Diamond DM, Hama R, *et al.* Lack of an association or an inverse association between low-density-lipoprotein cholesterol and mortality in the elderly: a systematic review. BMJ Open. 2016;6:e010401 https://bmjopen.bmj.com/content/bmjopen/6/6/e010401.full.pdf

4. Diamond DM, Ravnskov U. How statistical deception created the appearance that statins are safe and effective in primary and secondary prevention of cardiovascular disease. Expert Rev Clin Pharmacol. 2015;8:201–210. https://tinyurl.se/1zV

5. Ravnskov U, de Lorgeril M, Kendrick M, Diamond DM. Inborn coagulation factors are more important cardiovascular risk factors than high LDL-cholesterol in familial hypercholesterolemia. Med Hypotheses 2018;121:60-3. https://tinyurl.se/1zW

Why do Statins Show no Benefits in Japan?

Tomohito Hamazaki MD, Phd, Harumi Okuyama Phd, Paul J. Rosch MD

Abstract

Recent Japanese epidemiological studies have shown no relationship between blood cholesterol levels and coronary heart disease (CHD) or all-cause mortality. Some Japanese researchers claim that the increasing and widespread use of statins over the past two decades has reduced CHD mortality to such an extent, that this data can no longer be utilized to establish cholesterol guidelines and should be replaced by CHD development statistics. On the other hand, if statins were so effective in reducing CHD mortality, then they should have a similar effect on CHD development, which would also impair using this to establish meaningful Japanese cholesterol guidelines. We question whether statins reduce CHD or total mortality. The primary prevention of cardiovascular disease with pravastatin in Japan (MEGA Study) is the only prospective randomized controlled statin trial that is available. It was designed to assess whether evidence for treatment with statins derived from western countries can be extrapolated to Japan, but as will be seen, it has several flaws. There is no reliable data to support the belief that statins prolong life in Japan, and since the Japanese have already succeeded in preventing CHD without decreasing cholesterol levels, their focus should be on something else.

1. Why Do Japanese With High Cholesterol or LDL Live Longer?

1.1 Older Japanese studies showed that people with high cholesterol levels live longer

As previously noted, all-cause mortality of Japanese people with

127

elevated cholesterol or LDL-cholesterol levels is low, compared to controls with low cholesterol levels.[1] The Ibaraki Prefectural Health Study,[2] a large epidemiological survey also confirms this, as can be seen in Fig. 1. The only Japanese report that found a correlation between cholesterol and all-cause mortality was the 2007 NIPPON DATA80 (ND80) study,[3] in which the highest total cholesterol levels (≥260 mg/dL or ≥6.71 mmol/L) were associated with the highest all-cause mortality, as shown in Fig. 2 below.

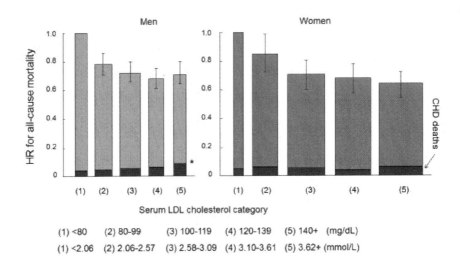

FIGURE 1 **Relationship Between Serum LDL-cholesterol Levels And The Hazard Ratio For All-cause Mortality In The Ibaraki Prefecture Study2**

In total, 30,802 men and 60,417 women were followed up for a median of 10.3 years. Hazard ratios (HRs) of all-cause mortality were adjusted for age and 11 other potential confounding factors. Darker colors show deaths from coronary heart disease (CHD). The height of the bar for deaths from CHD is set according to the ratio of the number of deaths from CHD to the number of all-cause deaths in the respective group. The phenomenon shown – that people with high cholesterol levels live longer than those with low cholesterol levels – can be explained by reverse causality; in other words, participants with high cholesterol levels lived longer because some participants with lower cholesterol levels due to a serious disease that was not yet known (e.g., hidden cancer) died early in the study period. To exclude the possibility of reverse causality, data were re-analyzed to exclude deaths that occurred within the first 2 years after baseline measurement. Interestingly, this did not substantially change the initial

results, indicating that effects of reverse causality were small. Vertical lines indicate 95% confidence intervals.
: Significantly different (p < 0.05) from the reference group (< 80 mg/dL) with regard to deaths from CHD. The width of each column is proportional to the number of participants in that group.

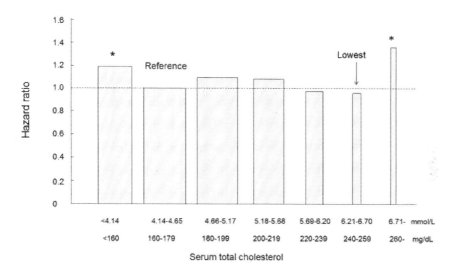

FIGURE 2 **Hazard Ratio For All-cause Mortality In Relation To Serum Total Cholesterol Levels**

*In total, 9216 participants (4035 men and 5181 women) were followed up for 17.3 years. Hazard ratios for all-cause mortality were adjusted for age, sex, body mass index, serum albumin levels, hypertension, diabetes, smoking habit, and drinking habit. However, the group with the highest cholesterol levels also contained an unusually large number of participants with familial hypercholesterolemia (see text). *: Significantly different from the reference group (p < 0.05). The width of each column is proportional to the number of participants in that group. See also Table 1 for details. The figure was drawn by us using the data in Table 2 from one[3] of the NIPPON DATA80 papers with permission.*

However, we must be very careful when interpreting the findings of NIPPON DATA80 because the study had several flaws (Table 1). For example, as we can see in Fig. 2, the hazard ratio for all-cause mortality was highest in the group with the highest total cholesterol levels (> 260 mg/dL, > 6.71 mmol/L). So, why did this conflicting result occur in the NIPPON DATA80 study? We need to consider familial hypercholesterolemia (FH) specifically here. FH is an inherited genetic disorder that is characterized by high LDL-cholesterol levels and early cardiovascular disease. In NIPPON DATA80, the highest number of deaths from any cause in the highest cholesterol group can be explained by this group theoretically containing most of the study participants with FH in the study. Moreover, the study involved nearly 3 times as many men with FH and 1.5 times as many women with FH than people in the general Japanese population with FH.[1]

It is also important to note that when an association is found between factors, such as between the highest cholesterol level and the number of deaths in this case, this does not mean that there is a causative relationship between them. Other research has linked LDL receptor disorder that occurs in FH with coagulation factors, inflammatory tone through tumor necrosis factor-α, and infectivity through complement C9 because the LDL receptor is a mosaic protein composed of exons shared with different proteins.[4] Also, coagulation factors are known to be more important cardiovascular risk factors in FH than high LDL cholesterol levels,[5] and cholesterol levels have been successfully decreased only in an animal experiment using the drug probucol, which has also anticoagulant effects, is not a statin, and was temporarily withdrawn from the market for safety reasons.[5] Some of the flaws in NIPPON DATA 80 are listed in Table 1.

On the whole then, Japanese epidemiological studies indicate that we should not view cholesterol as an enemy but rather as a good friend.[1] How can we explain the low all-cause mortality in people with high cholesterol levels? An answer could be suggested by the findings of another Japanese epidemiological study, the Isehara Study.[6] Interestingly, Fig. 3 shows that the top LDL-cholesterol group among men (panel A) and among women (panel B) in the study had only roughly one third to one half of the deaths from respiratory disease (light gray columns) compared with such deaths in all other LDL cholesterol groups. Respiratory disease comprised mostly deaths from pneumonia (because lung cancer was included under deaths from malignancy [black columns]), so probably one of the best candidates to explain the causal relationship is the neutralizing effects of LDL particles against toxic microorganisms and their debris.[1, 7] In addition, reverse causality (see legend to Fig. 1) could not explain here because pneumonia appeared years after cholesterol measurement, not before.

1 More FH participants were included in the study than in the general Japanese population	Nearly 3 times more in men and 1.5 times in women. In this way cholesterol can be impressed as poison.[1]
2 Data were adjusted for serum albumin levels	This adjustment attenuated cholesterol's beneficial effects because there is a highly significant correlation between cholesterol and albumin levels (over-adjustment). Cholesterol not only indicates nutrition levels like albumin but works as the first defense line against infectious agents and their debris, which albumin can hardly fulfill.[1]
3 In the original Figure 1 in the ND80 paper[3] sex-adjusted allcause mortality was shown.	If shown according to sex, the significantly increased mortality did not appear except for two male groups of total cholesterol levels <160 and 200-219 mg/dl (<4.14 mmol/L and 5.18-5.68 mmol/L, respectively) compared with the control (160-179 mg/dl, 4.14-4.65 mmol/L).
4 Participants were recruited from 300 small districts all over Japan; besides ND80 expressed their research focus on circulatory-disease.	This procedure might reduce area-specific biases, but failed in gathering average Japanese participants. The mean number of participants per area was only 35; more participants with circulatory problems, FH for example, were recruited. This type of error was almost completely nullified in the case of the Ibaraki Prefecture Health Study, which recruited participants from a whole prefecture (Ibaraki Prefecture).

TABLE 1 The list of flaws found in NIPPON DATA80*

---

* See also Fig. 2 for NIPPON DATA80.

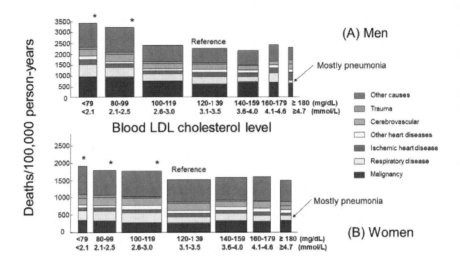

FIGURE 3 Relationship Between LDL Cholesterol Levels And The Number of Deaths In (A) Men and (B) Women In The Isehara Study[6]

In total, 8,340 male (aged 64 ± 10 years) and 13,591 female (61 ± 12 years) residents in Isehara City, Japan, were followed over 11 years for a mean follow-up period of 7.1 years (1994-2004) using the city's health check-up system. Deaths during the first year of follow up were excluded to account for the possibility of reverse causality. Cox's proportional hazards regression analysis was used to calculate age-adjusted relative risks.
*: p < 0.001 with Bonferroni adjustment. The width of each column is proportional to the number of participants in that group. Reproduced with permission from Ann Nutr Metab 2015;66 Suppl 4:1-1161 (Fig. 1-2).

1.2 Why recent Japanese studies fail to include cholesterol or LDL and total mortality data

Except for a 2014 study conducted in Fukuoka, Japan,[8] recent Japanese studies published between 2014 and 2019[9-12] have not reported any relationship between serum cholesterol levels (total, LDL, or non-HDL) and deaths from any cause or deaths from CHD. Why hasn't any such data been reported in recent Japanese studies? A comment from Makoto Kinoshita, the chairperson of the Preparation Committee of Japan Atherosclerosis Society (JAS) Guidelines for Prevention of Atherosclerotic Cardiovascular Diseases 2017,[13] which

132

appeared in *Medical Tribune* (a Japanese medical news journal, Issue of September 4th, 2017), may explain what has been happening. Our translation of his comment into English, which uses the terms "coronary artery disease" (CAD) and "CHD" interchangeably, is as follows:

"The previous [JAS] guidelines had been using the cohort study [NIPPON DATA80],[3] which investigated the risks of death from coronary artery disease (CAD), as the mainstay reference for evaluating such risks. However, the common use of statins in the recent years has reduced the number of deaths from CAD, and we thought that we should attach importance to CHD development rather than to CAD deaths".

This comment may seem logical at first, but is obviously inconsistent. If deaths from CAD (or CHD) are being reduced by people taking statins (which is actually wrong, especially in Japan; see Section 2 below), then there should also be fewer people developing CAD, and none of the statin-contaminated epidemiological studies – which is essentially all recent studies – should be referred to when evaluating the relationship between serum cholesterol levels and development of CHD. One[11] of the Suita study reports, which was published in 2014, was used as the main reference for the JAS Guidelines for Prevention of Atherosclerotic Cardiovascular Diseases 2017,[13] and it presented risk factors for CHD calculated with data from 213 CHD cases (not deaths). Unconventionally, the report did not present any details of the 213 cases such as the male to female ratio, number of deaths, or age at death, and there was no information about the relationship between cholesterol levels and deaths from any cause, despite the date and even time of each death being meticulously recorded.[11] As we reported previously,[1] we had been studying the references used to develop all versions of the JAS Guidelines published before the 2017 version, and we found the basis for the 2017 version, the Suita study,[11] was no better than the previous fragile bases for the earlier JAS guidelines. (For more information about flaws in the Suita study,[11] see our report although with an English abstract only.[14])

133

1.3 Investigators should disclose data on the relationship between cholesterol and deaths

If statins are indeed so effective that they reduce deaths from CHD or from any cause (thereby obfuscating the data on deaths in epidemiological studies), the researchers conducting these studies – which they are ethically responsible for reporting properly – should disclose any data they have on the relationship between cholesterol and deaths from any cause. Not publishing important data is a betrayal of the study participants. Most researchers involved in this area of work supposedly believe that cholesterol is, without a doubt, a serious risk for CHD and that statins are the drug of choice. The fact that participants with the highest cholesterol levels survived longer than participants in other cholesterol groups offers researchers the perfect chance to prove their notion that statins are effective at reducing deaths. So why aren't they publishing the data to support their notion?

But can statins actually reduce deaths of any kind? In Section 2, we explain that statins have never been proven to prolong life span; on the contrary, they are very likely to shorten it, especially in Japan.

2. Do statins shorten life span in Japan?

2.1 Brief Introduction to the MEGA Study

Kristensen *et al.*[15] estimated how long statins postponed death using data from 6 controlled statin trials for primary prevention and 5 for secondary prevention (Table 2), all of which provided a Kaplan-Meier plot of deaths from any cause. Death was postponed between −5 and 19 days with a median of 3.2 days with statins for primary prevention and between −10 and 27 days with a median of 4.1 days with statins for secondary prevention. According to our own calculations, it should be noted that neither of the median postponed periods was significantly different from the null value. One of the 6 trials on primary prevention is a paper from Japan, the MEGA Study.16 In this section, we discuss the MEGA Study because it also had several serious flaws, and because it is recognized as the only randomized controlled statin trial in Japan – actually it was only apparently randomized – and so it has substantially influenced clinical practice in Japan. Indeed, this trial has been cited as the major reference work in all of the recent JAS treatment guidelines.[1]

Study ID (Publication Year)	Intervention/ comparator	Postponement of deaths (days)	Number of participants after randomization Group		Difference
			Placebo/ usual care	Statin	
WOSCOPS 1995	Prava/pl*	9.33	3293	3302	-9
ALLHAT-LLT 2002	Prava/uc*	-4.96	5185	5170	15
ASCOT-LLA 2003	Atorva/pl	1.99	5137	5168	-31
CARDS 2004	Atorva/pl	18.66	1410	1428	-18
JUPITER 2008	Rosuva/pl	7.26	8901	8901	0
MEGA 2006	Prava/nt*	4.42	3966	3866	**100**

TABLE 2 **Postponement of death by statins (primary prevention) and difference in numbers of participants between active and control groups**

Data were collected from Kristensen et al.'s paper15 with intervention trials listed in the left column. See text for explanation of the right column.
* pl=placebo, uc=usual care, nt=no treatment

The MEGA Study,[16] recognized as a prospective, randomised, open-labelled, blinded endpoint (PROBE) study, recruited patients with hypercholesterolemia and no history of CHD or stroke. A profile of the Study is shown in Fig. 4. The participants were assigned either to diet or to diet plus pravastatin daily. Mean follow-up was 5.3 years. The primary endpoint, which was the first occurrence of CHD including fatal and non-fatal myocardial infarction, angina, cardiac and sudden death, and a coronary revascularization procedure, was significantly lower in the diet plus pravastatin group than in the diet alone group (HR 0.67, 95% CI, 0.49-0.91; p = 0.01).

2.2 Serious flaws in the MEGA Study

The MEGA Study[16] should not have been cited in the Kristensen *et al* .paper, which was limited to a discussion of only randomized trials.[15] Postponement of death in the study was calculated to be 4.42 days according to their paper.[15] Actually all-cause mortality was lower in the statin plus diet group (2.7/1000 person-years, 55 deaths) than in the control (diet only) group (3.8/1000, 79 deaths) with marginal significance, the hazard ratio being 0.72 (0.51–1.01, P=0.055).[16] These results were amazing, considering that total mortality can hardly be significantly improved by statin therapy even in secondary prevention trials. The Scandinavian Simvastatin Survival Study (4S)[17] is probably the rarest exception in secondary prevention.

How were these magnificent results obtained in the MEGA Study, particularly in primary prevention? The answer is partially clarified in Fig. 4. In the MEGA Study, 3966 participants were assigned to the diet alone group, and 3866 to the diet plus statin group. Consequently, 100 more participants were excluded from the statin group AFTER randomization. Figure 1 of the original paper[16] (Fig. 4 below) is so ambiguous, it is not immediately clear if randomization was performed before or after the exclusion of 382 participants. The details of exclusion were: 94 without consent, 224 exclusion criteria violation, and 64 no recorded data AFTER randomization (see Fig. 4). (The two emphases "AFTER"s above are by us.) The phrase in Fig. 4 "64 no recorded data after randomization" definitely indicates that arrows in the flow chart (Fig. 4) are set in wrong places; the bifurcation arrows, which usually point where randomization took place, should have been placed right below the box of "8214 patients randomized".

See the red arrow. It seems that 100 more participants were excluded from the diet plus statin group than from the diet alone group. Reproduced with permission from the original paper[16] with truncation and slight modifications (originally Figure 1).

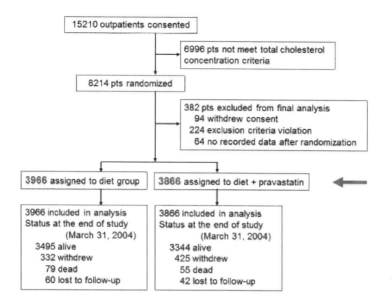

```
┌──────────────────────────────┐
│ 15210 outpatients consented   │
└──────────────────────────────┘
                │        ┌────────────────────────────────────┐
                ├───────▶│ 6996 pts not meet total cholesterol │
                │        │ concentration criteria              │
                │        └────────────────────────────────────┘
┌──────────────────────────┐
│ 8214 pts randomized        │
└──────────────────────────┘
                │        ┌─────────────────────────────────────────────┐
                ├───────▶│ 382 pts excluded from final analysis        │
                │        │    94 withdrew consent                      │
                │        │   224 exclusion criteria violation          │
                │        │    64 no recorded data after randomization  │
                │        └─────────────────────────────────────────────┘
     ┌──────────┴──────────┐
     ▼                     ▼
```

| 3966 assigned to diet group | 3866 assigned to diet + pravastatin | ◀━━━━ |

3966 included in analysis	3866 included in analysis
Status at the end of study	Status at the end of study
(March 31, 2004)	(March 31, 2004)
3495 alive	3344 alive
332 withdrew	425 withdrew
79 dead	55 dead
60 lost to follow-up	42 lost to follow-up

FIGURE 4 **Profile of The Mega Study (Management of Elevated Cholesterol in the Primary Prevention Group of Adult Japanese)**

2.3 The fact that the MEGA Study wanted to hide

If 8214 participants had been randomly divided into two groups, each group would have had 4107 participants. The readers can easily understand how strange this 100 difference between groups is by scanning and comparing the differences of the other five primary prevention trials introduced by Kristensen et al.[15] (see last column of Table 2). The differences of those five trials were scattered in the narrow range of −31 and 15 participants. If those differences were very large, especially if more participants were excluded from the treatment group than from controls, as in the MEGA study, one might suspect that unfavorable participants for the trial had been excluded from the treatment group. In order to prevent such suspicions, researchers conducting randomized clinical trials would presumably like to make such differences as small as possible. The method is simple enough; just divide the whole participants randomly into two groups. This simple and clear rule did not work for the MEGA study, so why did the authors disregard this?

Found flaw	Comments
1 In the figure (Figure 3 of the original MEGA Study paper[16]) showing the relation between CHD incident (%) against time (up to 6 years), a completely straight horizontal line of about 13 months, which means no CHD events were reported at all, was reported in the statin group near the end of the trial.	The possibility of appearance of such a straight line was calculated as p<0.01. The study period was originally planned to be 5 years, but elongated to more than 6. The straight line just started to appear when the study plan was revised and the study populations of both groups dropped suddenly. Unfavorable (unhealthy) participants were highly likely not asked to remain in the statin group of the Study, so that randomization was again destroyed.
2 The primary endpoint was a composite endpoint including fatal and non-fatal myocardial infarction, angina, cardiac and sudden death, and coronary revascularization.	Diagnosis of composite endpoint is known to be biased in favor of the test drug. The composite endpoint of the MEGA Study included "angina" and "coronary revascularization", which are easily determined in a non-objective way and not reliable.
3 Participants in both groups were placed on an alleged cholesterol-lowering diet. However, cholesterol levels hardly changed in the diet alone group, and more participants in this group adhered to the diet.	The diet used in the Study was old fashioned. Butter was replaced with margarine containing a lot of linoleic acid and/or trans fatty acids, and fatty fish was avoided because it contained too much cholesterol. Very unfortunately, this diet was CHD inducing. Due to decreased cholesterol levels, participants in the diet plus statin group did not stick to the diet. Decreased CHD incidence in the statin group was ironically not because of statin use but of weak compliance to that diet.

TABLE 3 **Serious flaws in the MEGA Study,[16] the only controlled Japanese statin study**

The answer may be that they wanted to conceal certain data. Before its *Lancet* 2006 publication[16], the MEGA Study had been orally presented at the 2005 American Heart Association Scientific Sessions. Hama *et al.*[18] later discussed the presentation using a Japanese version of a MEGA study set of slides. This revealed that 13.5% of participants could not be confirmed to be alive in the pravastatin plus diet group, but that such participants were 11.9% in the diet alone group (odds ratio: 1.16, 1.01-1.33, p=0.031).[1] The authors might not have wanted to mention this, and we presume that they decided to exclude unfavorable participants from the statin group instead. In addition to this dubious randomization, the MEGA study contained other serious flaws as listed in Table 3 below. Consequently, the present authors do not fully understand the results of the Study, especially those of all-cause mortality.

3. CHD mortality and FH in Japan

If all-cause mortality increases in people taking statins as previously indicated, large-scale epidemiological studies should find that the lower cholesterol levels are, the longer you will live, since people with high cholesterol levels were more likely to take statins, and therefore might die more frequently, which might be misconstrued as supporting the cholesterol hypothesis. However, it is more likely that the opposite occurs.

In some FH participants, thrombosis-prone coagulation factor gene(s) are co-inherited as described above, and a sizable portion of these individuals die relatively sooner after the start of epidemiological studies leaving only thrombosis-resistant FH participants. As a result, seemingly unfavorable effects of high cholesterol found in these individuals will fade over time.[1, 19] This phenomenon is not limited to Japan since it is seen all over the world.[20] The 2014 Fukuoka study is a typical example.[8] Japanese participants, who were essentially free from thrombosis-prone FH because they were all 85 years old, were followed for 10 years. All-cause mortality against total cholesterol tertiles revealed that the total mortality in the low-cholesterol group was 1.7-fold higher than that in the high-cholesterol group after adjustment for eight confounding factors. The influence of decreasing numbers of thrombosis-prone FH seems to be much stronger in epidemiological studies, than mortality due to statin use.

Conclusion

CHD mortality in Japan has been very low compared to other well developed coutries,[21] and accounts only for one seventh of all Japanese deaths. This preventive effect is not related to lipid effects, since mean cholesterol levels are not low[22] and have been increasing. Considering the very few cases of CHD, it is understandable that proving any efficacy of statins or other cholesterol lowering drugs, must be tremendously difficult without ludicrous and absurd methods of pseudo-randomization. We can also cite the Kyushu Lipid Intervention Study as another pseudo-randomization trial[23] (for details see our paper[1]). As a result, recent epidemiological studies cannot provide accurate information on CHD mortality, but only on its development.

So, what explains the surprisingly low CHD mortality in Japan? We suggest that the focus should be shifted from cholesterol and LDL to something else, such as omega-3 rich fish oil, which contains DHA (docosahexaenoic acid) and EPA (eicosapentaenoic acid). These omega-3 fats, are very likely to reduce coronary calcification and calcium density in Japanese men, and coronary atherosclerosis in the general population,[24] reduce the risk of sudden cardiac death and fatal coronary events,[25] reduce the risk of metabolic syndrome[26] reduce inflammation and cardiovascular disease,[27-29] improve rheumatoid arthritis,[30] lower blood pressure.[31] Those fats, especially DHA, are important for brain growth and function and may prevent or delay the onset of Alzheimer's,[32, 33] improve endothelial function and lower risk for colorectal, pancreatic, breast and prostate cancers and improve chemotherapy results.[34-37] They have numerous other benefits,[38] one of the most important being reducing stress. As explained in another chapter in this book, stress is a major cause of coronary heart disease,[39] and omega-3 fatty acids have proved effective in preventing and treating depression.[40] In addition, supplementing DHA to Japanese students, who do not eat fish very often, was shown to control stressor-induced behavior changes such as aggression prior to term or final exams, as was demonstrated in a double-blind study.[41]

The cholesterol obituary should have been written long ago, and while the above is just another nail in the coffin, it suggests there might be something to replace it.

Tomohito Hamazaki* MD, PhD, Harumi Okuyama** PhD, Paul J. Rosch** MD

*Emeritus Professor, Toyama University, and Toyama Jonan Onsen Daini Hospital, 1-13-6 Taromaru-Nishimachi, Toyama-City, Toyama 939-8271, Japan

** Professor Emeritus, Nagoya City University, and Institute for Consumer Science and Human Life, Kinjo Gakuin University, 2-1723 Omori, Moriyama, Nagoya 463-8521, Japan

*** Clinical Professor of Medicine and Psychiatry, New York Medical College, Valhalla, NY, USA and Chairman, The American Institute of Stress, Weatherford TX, USA

References

1. Hamazaki T, Okuyama H, Ogushi Y, Hama R. Towards a Paradigm Shift in Cholesterol Treatment. A Re-examination of the Cholesterol Issue in Japan. Ann Nutr Metab 2015;66 Suppl 4:1-116.

2. Noda H, Iso H, Irie F, Sairenchi T, Ohtaka E, Ohta H. Gender difference of association between LDL cholesterol concentrations and mortality from coronary heart disease amongst Japanese: the Ibaraki Prefectural Health Study. J Intern Med 2010;267:576-87.

3. Okamura T, Tanaka H, Miyamatsu N, *et al.* The relationship between serum total cholesterol and all-cause or cause-specific mortality in a 17.3-year study of a Japanese cohort. Atherosclerosis 2007;190:216-23.

4. Sudhof TC, Goldstein JL, Brown MS, Russell DW. The LDL receptor gene: a mosaic of exons shared with different proteins. Science 1985;228:815-22.

5. Ravnskov U, de Lorgeril M, Kendrick M, Diamond DM. Inborn coagulation factors are more important cardiovascular risk factors than high LDL-cholesterol in familial hypercholesterolemia. Med Hypotheses 2018;121:60-3.

6. Ogushi Y, Kurita Y. Resident cohort study to analyze relations between health check-up results and cause-specific mortality. Mumps (M Technology Association Japan) 2008;24:9-19 (in Japanese).

7. Ravnskov U, McCully KS. Review and Hypothesis: Vulnerable plaque formation from obstruction of Vasa vasorum by homocysteinylated and oxidized lipoprotein aggregates complexed with microbial remnants and LDL autoantibodies. Ann Clin Lab Sci 2009;39:3-16.

141

8. Takata Y, Ansai T, Soh I, *et al.* Serum total cholesterol concentration and 10-year mortality in an 85-year-old population. Clin Interv Aging 2014;9:293-300.

9. Hirata T, Sugiyama D, Nagasawa SY, *et al.* A pooled analysis of the association of isolated low levels of high-density lipoprotein cholesterol with cardiovascular mortality in Japan. Eur J Epidemiol 2017;32:547-57.

10. Ito T, Arima H, Fujiyoshi A, *et al.* Relationship between non-high-density lipoprotein cholesterol and the long-term mortality of cardiovascular diseases: NIPPON DATA 90. Int J Cardiol 2016;220:262-7.

11. Nishimura K, Okamura T, Watanabe M, *et al.* Predicting coronary heart disease using risk factor categories for a Japanese urban population, and comparison with the Framingham risk score: the Suita study. J Atheroscler Thromb 2014;21:784-98.

12. Shibata Y, Ojima T, Nakamura M, *et al.* Associations of Overweight, Obesity, and Underweight With High Serum Total Cholesterol Level Over 30 Years Among the Japanese Elderly: NIPPON DATA 80, 90, and 2010. J Epidemiol 2019;29:133-8.

13. Japan Atherosclerosis Society. Japan Atherosclerosis Society (JAS) Guidelines for Prevention of Atherosclerotic Cardiovascular Diseases 2017 (in Japanese). Ed by Japan Atherosclerosis Society 2017.

14. Okuyama H, Kasamoto S, Hamazaki T. Mechanisms of atherogenesis without involving elevated LDL-cholesterol, and critical evaluation of the Japan Atherosclerosis Society Guidelines for Prevention of Atherosclerotic Cardiovascular Diseases 2017. J Lipid Nutr 2018;27:21-9 (with English abstract).

15. Kristensen ML, Christensen PM, Hallas J. The effect of statins on average survival in randomised trials, an analysis of end point postponement. BMJ Open 2015;5:e007118.

16. Nakamura H, Arakawa K, Itakura H, *et al.* Primary prevention of cardiovascular disease with pravastatin in Japan (MEGA Study): a prospective randomised controlled trial. *Lancet* 2006;368:1155-63.

17. Scandinavian Simvastatin Survival Study Group. Randomised trial of cholesterol lowering in 4444 patients with coronary heart disease: the Scandinavian Simvastatin Survival Study (4S). *Lancet* 1994;344:1383-9.

18. Hama R, Sakaguchi K. Pravastatin (mevalotin) reduces survival rates – a critical examination on MEGA Study – NNTH 48: Administration of pravastatin to 48 subjects for 5.3 years reduces one survivor. Informed Prescriber 2006;21:84-6 (in Japanese).

19. Okuyama H, Hamazaki T, Ogushi Y, al e. Cholesterol guidelines for longevity, 2010, ed by Japan Society for Lipid Nutrition (in Japanese). Chunichi Shuppansha, Nagoya-city 2010

20. Ravnskov U, Diamond DM, Hama R, *et al.* Lack of an association or an inverse association between low-density-lipoprotein cholesterol and mortality in the elderly: a systematic review. BMJ Open 2016;6:e010401.

21. Finegold JA, Asaria P, Francis DP. Mortality from ischaemic heart disease by country, region, and age: statistics from World Health Organisation and United Nations. Int J Cardiol 2013;168:934-45.

22. Global Health Observatory data repository. Mean total cholesterol trends (age-standardized estimate). Data by country. http://appswhoint/gho/data/viewmain12469.

23. The Kyushu Lipid Intervention Study Group. Pravastatin use and risk of coronary events and cerebral infarction in Japanese men with moderate hypercholesterolemia: the Kyushu Lipid Intervention Study. J Atheroscler Thromb 2000;7:110-21.

24. Sekikawa A, Mahajan H, Kadowaki S, *et al.* Association of blood levels of marine omega-3 fatty acids with coronary calcification and calcium density in Japanese men. Eur J Clin Nutr 2019;73:783-92.

25. Hamazaki K, Iso H, Eshak ES, *et al.* Plasma levels of n-3 fatty acids and risk of coronary heart disease among Japanese: The Japan Public Health Center-based (JPHC) study. Atherosclerosis 2018;272:226-32.

26. Guo XF, Li X, Shi M, Li D. n-3 Polyunsaturated Fatty Acids and Metabolic Syndrome Risk: A Meta-Analysis. Nutrients 2017;9.

27. Allaire J, Couture P, Leclerc M, *et al.* A randomized, crossover, head-to-head comparison of eicosapentaenoic acid and docosahexaenoic acid supplementation to reduce inflammation markers in men and women: the Comparing EPA to DHA (CompareD) Study. Am J Clin Nutr 2016;104:280-7.

28. Tabbaa M, Golubic M, Roizen MF, Bernstein AM. Docosahexaenoic acid, inflammation, and bacterial dysbiosis in relation to periodontal disease, inflammatory bowel disease, and the metabolic syndrome. Nutrients 2013;5:3299-310.

29. Schunck WH, Konkel A, Fischer R, Weylandt KH. Therapeutic potential of omega-3 fatty acid-derived epoxyeicosanoids in cardiovascular and inflammatory diseases. Pharmacol Ther 2018;183:177-204.

30. Dawczynski C, Dittrich M, Neumann T, *et al.* Docosahexaenoic acid in the treatment of rheumatoid arthritis: A double-blind, placebo-controlled, randomized cross-over study with microalgae vs. sunflower oil. Clin Nutr 2018;37:494-504.

31. Guo XF, Li KL, Li JM, Li D. Effects of EPA and DHA on blood pressure and inflammatory factors: a meta-analysis of randomized controlled trials. Crit Rev Food Sci Nutr 2019:1-14.

32. Kuratko CN, Barrett EC, Nelson EB, Salem N, Jr. The relationship of docosahexaenoic acid (DHA) with learning and behavior in healthy children: a review. Nutrients 2013;5:2777-810.

33. Yanai H. Effects of N-3 Polyunsaturated Fatty Acids on Dementia. J Clin Med Res 2017;9:1-9.

34. Ortea I, Gonzalez-Fernandez MJ, Ramos-Bueno RP, Guil-Guerrero JL. Proteomics Study Reveals That Docosahexaenoic and Arachidonic Acids Exert Different In Vitro Anticancer Activities in Colorectal Cancer Cells. J Agric Food Chem 2018;66:6003-12.

35. Yum HW, Na HK, Surh YJ. Anti-inflammatory effects of docosahexaenoic acid: Implications for its cancer chemopreventive potential. Semin Cancer Biol 2016;40-41:141-59.

143

36. Newell M, Baker K, Postovit LM, Field CJ. A Critical Review on the Effect of Docosahexaenoic Acid (DHA) on Cancer Cell Cycle Progression. Int J Mol Sci 2017;18.

37. Song EA, Kim H. Docosahexaenoic Acid Induces Oxidative DNA Damage and Apoptosis, and Enhances the Chemosensitivity of Cancer Cells. Int J Mol Sci 2016;17.

38. Zarate R, El Jaber-Vazdekis N, Tejera N, Perez JA, Rodriguez C. Significance of long chain polyunsaturated fatty acids in human health. Clin Transl Med 2017;6:25.

39. Rosch PJ. The Crucial Role Of Stress In Coronary Heart Disease

40. McNamara RK. Role of Omega-3 Fatty Acids in the Etiology, Treatment, and Prevention of Depression: Current Status and Future Directions. J Nutr Intermed Metab 2016;5:96-106.

41. Hamazaki T, Sawazaki S, Itomura M, et al. The effect of docosahexaenoic acid on aggression in young adults. A placebo-controlled double-blind study. J Clin Invest 1996;97:1129-33.

Statins Can Cause Heart Failure and Increase Atherosclerosis and Coronary Artery Calcification

Harumi Okuyama PhD, Tomohito Hamazaki MD, PhD, Paul J. Rosch MD

Abstract

[1] Statins inhibit an early step of cholesterol synthesis, and reduce downstream products such as isopentenyl pyrophosphate (PP), geranyl PP, farnesyl PP etc. Farnesyl PP is necessary to synthesize heme A and utilized for CoQ10 and vitamin K2 production after its conversion to geranyl-geranyl PP. Heme A and CoQ10 are indispensable components of the electron transport system in the mitochondrion. Statins has thus mitochondrion-toxic effects.

[2] Although randomized controlled trials indicate statins have no effects on heart failure (HF) mortality, statin's adverse effects become apparent if focused on very ill patients who might be already depleted of CoQ10. The HF incidence in Japan has been actually increasing faster than the ageing speed of the Japanese population despite statin prevalence. Keshan disease, congestive HF seen in selenium (Se)-deficient soil areas, may somehow be similar to statin's adverse effects, because statins inhibit isopentenyl PP, which is a necessary part of tRNAsc, transporter of selenocysteine. Selenoproteins involve glutathione peroxidase, iodothyronine deiodinase, thioredoxin reductases and some other important proteins. Consequently, statins may cause HF even without anti-mitochondrion effects.

[3] Statins decrease vitamin K2 levels through shortening of geranyl-geranyl PP and inhibiting prenyltransferase activity, which leads to γ-carboxylated gla-protein deficiency and thereby soft tissue calcification. Indeed, coronary artery calcification (CAC) in statin users is shown both in cross-sectional and intervention studies. Some researchers insist that CAC without statins is bad, and CAC with statins is good, but this argument seems opportunistic.

145

1. Statins are toxic to mitochondria and can cause heart failure

Statins decrease important components in mitochondria and disturb the anti-oxidative enzyme system necessary for mitochondrial integrity. These effects explain disorders of mitochondrion-rich organs by statins, namely, muscles, including the heart.

1-1. What biomaterials can statins decrease in addition to cholesterol?

At first, we need to elucidate what step in cholesterol synthesis is stopped by statins. Fig. 1 is a simplified pathway of cholesterol and prenyl intermediate biosynthesis. Actually, there are some 30 steps to complete cholesterol synthesis. The starting substrate of cholesterol is acetyl-coenzyme A (CoA). After a couple of enzymatic actions, acetyl-CoA becomes 3-hydroxy-3-methylglutaryl-CoA (HMG-CoA), which is reduced to mevalonic acid. This is the very step where statins, in other words HMG-CoA reductase inhibitors, can inhibit, which means that all the biomaterials produced downstream are also decreased due to the absence of any tributary to the mainstream. Indispensable biomaterials called prenyl intermediates are found downstream. Geranyl and farnesyl compounds are two examples.

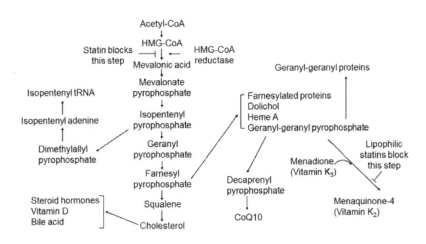

FIGURE 1 **Metabolic pathways of acetyl-CoA to cholesterol and prenyl intermediates**

146

1-2. Indispensable components of mitochondria containing prenyl intermediates

All physical movements and many enzymatic actions need ATP as their source of energy. The most important role of oxygen is to help produce ATP in mitochondria. The burning of sugar and fatty acids extracts hydrogen atom (H), which is divided into proton (H+) and electron (e-). e- is transported by way of the electron transport system in which complex I or II, coenzyme Q10 (CoQ10), complex III and complex IV are involved in this order (Fig. 2). Protons are gathered in the mitochondrial inter-membrane space (between outer- and inner-membranes), and high concentrations of H propel ATP synthase to create ATP. The point to take note here is that CoQ10 and heme A are also necessary components to transport e-. As shown in Fig. 1, these components include prenyl-intermediates in their molecules. Thus, statins depress mitochondrial CoQ10 and heme A contents, and can result in ATP deficiency. CoQ10 is abundantly contained in food, and consequently, CoQ10 deficiency is rare in healthy people, but it may happen in poorly nourished patients under statin treatment as shown below. CoQ10 exists in two redox forms. One of these reduced form (ubiquinol) is a clinically relevant antioxidant in the mitochondrial membranes. Mitochondrial DNA is more vulnerable to oxidative stress than nuclear DNA. Without the reduced form, mitochondrial DNA may be easily damaged.[1]

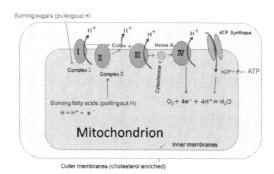

FIGURE 2 **Statins are mitochondrial toxins**

CoQ10 and Heme A are indispensable parts of the electron transportation system in mitochondria. Both have prenyl intermediate side chains. So, statins deteriorate ATP production, which may result in muscle aching and heart failure (see text). CoQ10 is also an important cofactor at other cellular metabolic steps.[2] Reproduced from figure 2 of reference 1.

Qu *et al.*[3], by meta-analyzing 12 randomized controlled statin trials, calculated blood CoQ10 levels and found a large reduction of blood CoQ10 (standardized mean difference, -2.12; 95% CI, -3.40 to -0.84; p = 0.001). The same group also evaluated the effects of CoQ10 on statin-induced myopathy through another metanalysis, and found that CoQ10 supplementation significantly ameliorated muscle symptoms such as pain, weakness, cramp, and tiredness.[4]

1-3. Can statins cause heart failure and death? (1)

Since statins harm mitochondria, can they easily deteriorate the cardiac functions of HF patients? Here we introduce two large heart failure-specific RCTs: CORONA[5] with 5011 HF patients aged ≥ 60 years, and the other GISSI-HF[6] with 4574 HF patients aged not less than 18 years. The daily dose of 10 mg rosuvastatin was used in the active groups in both trials. The all-cause mortality in CORONA trial was 29% and 30% (our calculation without adjustment) in the rosuvastatin and placebo groups, respectively, during a median follow-up of 32.8 months, and that of the GISSI-HF was similarly 29% and 28% during a median of 3.9 years.

In a recent study performed by Chin *et al.*[7] to determine the ability of statins to improve clinical outcomes among HF patients undergoing percutaneous coronary intervention (PCI), 991 patients were followed from 30 days to 1 year after PCI. Based on mean propensity scores, each statin-taking patient was matched to the most similar patients not taking a statin. The study found no significant effect of statins on the primary composite outcome (all-cause mortality and hospitalization for cardiovascular (CV) causes). The same was true for major adverse cardiac events and hospitalization for CV causes. It is important to comment on this. In their study, more dyslipidemia was found in patients taking statins than non-statin taking patients; namely, 78.2% vs. 60.0% (P<0.001). This must have favored the statin group. A considerable number of observational studies have indicated that lower cholesterol levels, total or LDL, are associated with less survival of chronic HF patients, and this association was attenuated by statin use but not eliminated.[8] Taking the above into account, an RCT administering statin or placebo to HF patients might result in poorer survival rates in the statin group under certain circumstances.

The 2015 meta-analysis paper of Preiss *et al.*[9] tried to establish statin effects on major HF events, and collected published and unpublished HF data from 21 RCTs. They did not find significant superiority of statin use for prevention of HF deaths, although the number of non-fatal HF hospitalization was significantly reduced (RR 0.90, 95% CI 0.84-0.97). However, hospitalization is not a hard endpoint because of introduction of bias, since doctors would know which patients were receiving statins to reduce cholesterol levels. As indicated in a previous paper[1], in order to correct (pharmaceutical industry-involved) mal-performance in clinical trials, new penal regulations took effect in 2004/2005. Since then, all clinical trials performed by researchers relatively free from conflict of interest, reported no significant beneficial effects of statins for the prevention of CHD. About two thirds of the papers cited by Preiss *et al.*[9] were before 2005 and, therefore, might not be as reliable.

It is highly likely that statins do not prevent serious outcomes of HF. However, we suggest that CoQ10 concentrations in the heart might be still well above the critical point in participants in those RCTs written above. If they were critically ill, they must have been excluded from trials. What if very ill patients are included in statin trials?

1-4. Can statins cause heart failure and death? (2)

We will discuss the following groups of extremely ill patients: 1. terminal patients with estimated survival period of 1-12 months (about one-half of them had cancer as their primary diagnosis), 2. those with acute respiratory distress syndrome (ARDS) at the immediate risk of other organ failure, and 3. those with ventilator-associated pneumonia. They might have suffered from CoQ10 depletion due to very poor nutrition and have the lowest levels of CoQ10 in various organs. In such situations, are statins harmful?

In cases of a short expected survival time,[10] all patients were on statin treatment for at least 3 months before the start of the trial, then they were randomly assigned to statin discontinuation or continuation. The death rate within 60 days, the primary endpoint, was 23.8%

in the discontinuation group and 20.3% in the continuation group (90%CI, −3.5% to 10.5%; p = 0.36). However, the survival curves were reversed just before 6 months, and a median time to death turned out to be 229 days (90% CI, 186–332) for the discontinuation and 190 days (90% CI, 170–257) for the continuation group (p = 0.60). Moreover, total quality of life and cost savings (secondary outcomes) were significantly better in the discontinuation group.

Regarding ARDS,[11] 1000 patients with sepsis-associated ARDS were scheduled to enter the trial. They were randomly assigned either to the rosuvastatin group or the placebo group. The primary endpoint was mortality before hospital discharge or day 60. One of the secondary endpoints was organ failure-free days to day 14. The trial was stopped after 745 patients were enrolled because of futility. No significant difference in mortality was found between the rosuvastatin group (28.5%) and the placebo group (24.9%, p = 0.21). Days free of renal failure were significantly reduced in the rosuvastatin group (10.1±5.3) compared with the placebo group (11.0±4.7, p= 0.01). Days free of hepatic failure were likewise decreased in the rosuvastatin group (10.8±5.0) compared with the placebo group (11.8±4.3, p = 0.003). In the case of ventilator-associated pneumonia,[12] originally 1002 patients were planned to enter a randomized trial to receive simvastatin or placebo. But this trial was also stopped after enrollment of 300 patients because mortality at day 28 was 21.2% in the simvastatin group compared with 15.2% in the placebo group (p = 0.10).

As shown above, two trials with serious infection failed in a row. The neutralizing effects of LDL against infectious organisms including endotoxins are well known (see Table 2-B of the reference[13]), and these effects may account for statin's failure in these infection-related trials. However, statin's toxic effects to mitochondria should also be considered, especially in the trial with ARDS, since significantly more frequent organ failures were noticed. Heart function was probably more damaged in statin groups as well. The point to make is the difference between CORONA[5]+GISSI-HF[6] and trials with seriously ill patients.[10-12] The conditions of the patients in the latter trials were so poor, their nutritional status including CoQ10 levels in tissues must have been at critical levels. As a result, patients in these three trials[10-12] were more likely to be vulnerable to the adverse effects of statins.

1-5. Why is heart failure increasing in Japan?

Heart failure (HF) has apparently been increasing in Japan. Fig. 3 shows the incidence of acute myocardial infarction (AMI) and HF from 2014 to 2018. Both AMI and HF have been increasing. Since ageing is probably the biggest risk factor of these diseases, we will discuss simplified trends of aging of the Japanese population and compare them with trends of both diseases. To begin, we focused on an age group of ≥ 65 years old in Japan, which includes a very large number of AMI and HF patients. Using a figure (Chart 1-1-2) included in Annual Report on the Ageing Society: 2018*, we estimated that the rate of increment of this age group was about 8.5%** in 4 years (between 2014 and 2018, the first and last years of Fig. 3).

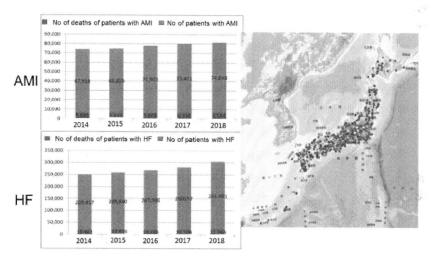

FIGURE 3 **The incidence of acute myocardial infarction and heart failure in the fixed observation hospitals in Japan**

Data were obtained from 1565 hospitals with departments of circulatory disease and/or cardiovascular surgery (see the map). Hospitals are: red, circulatory disease-specific teaching hospitals; blue, teaching hospitals; and yellow, others.

---

* Cabinet Office https://www8.cao.go.jp/kourei/english/annualreport/2018/2018pdf_e.html

** Details of calculation; the ratio of the population (aged ≥ 65) to the total population in Japan in 2014 was estimated to be 25.9%. That in 2018 was similarly 28.1. So, the rate of increment was 2.81/2.59 = 1.085 (8.5%).

151

Reproduced from figures found in JROAD (The Japanese Registry Of All cardiac and vascular Diseases) 2018; <http://www.j-circ.or.jp/jittai_chosa/#tensai>. Permission of reproduction is not required for academic use.

	Disease	Number of patients in the hospitals		% Increment of patients from	P values between % increments
		2014	2018	2014 to 2018	
Total number of in-patients	AMI	67,918	74,848	10.2%	P<0.0001
	HF	229,417	281,481	22.7%	
Number of in-patients deaths	AMI	5,838	6,564	12.4%	P=0.023
	HF	18,962	22,340	17.8%	

TABLE 1 The number of heart failure in the fixed observation hospitals in Japan is increasing

Numbers of patients were extracted from Fig. 3. Total number of beds in the registered hospitals did not barely change (545,042 and 545,426 in 2014 and 2018, respectively). The age group (≥ 65) in Japan was estimated to increase about 8.5 % from 2014 to 2018 (see previous page for explanation). AMI = acute myocardial infarction; HF = heart failure.
Reference for patient numbers: http://www.j-circ.or.jp/jittai_chosa/#tensai
Reference for population: https://www8.cao.go.jp/kourei/whitepaper/w2018/html/zenbun/s1_1_1.html

The data shown in Fig. 3 are of course not free from bias. Probably the most powerful bias might be the ageing of the Japanese population. The vulnerable age group (aged ≥ 65) increased only 8.5%, which allows us to presume that the increments of the AMI incidence (10.2%) and mortality (12.4%) in these 4 years of statin prevalence did not indicate any decreasing tendency in the fixed observation hospitals (Table 1). On the other hand, the HF incidence and mortality in the same settings has most likely being increasing because HF significantly increased more than AMI (Table 1).

In conclusion, according to the data from the fixed circulatory disease-specific hospitals (mostly teaching hospitals), which should be much more accurate than the whole data of the nation, HF has been increasing in Japan despite statin prevalence.

1-6. Keshan disease (Se-deficiency), a different type of heart failure, and a hint to understanding the adverse effects of statins

Keshan (the name of a province in China) disease is a congestive cardiomyopathy of those people who live in selenium (Se)-deficient soil areas. The disease, which is caused by a mutated strain of Coxsackievirus, and Se deficiency seems to induce a more virulent mutation of the virus.[14] Fortunately, supplementation with Se reduced the incidence of the disease over decades. Why are statins relevant to Keshan disease?

Se is incorporated into selenoproteins by the aid of tRNAsc, specific for transferring the Se-containing amino acid, selenocysteine. tRNAsc contains a minor base, isopentenyl adenine, which is synthesized with a prenyl-intermediate, isoprenyl pyrophosphate (see Fig. 1), and decreased by statins. The following enzymes are all selenoproteins: glutathione peroxidase, iodothyronine deiodinase, thioredoxin reductases etc. Although the following studies were animal experiments, they strongly suggest the relationship between Se-deficiency, glutathione peroxidase and virulence. In Se-deficient mice, a myocarditis-causing Coxsackievirus B3 genetically changed to a virulent strain. Similar alterations in virulence could be observed in glutathione peroxidase-knockout mice under normal diet.[14]

If peroxidative stress is elevated by inhibition of peroxidase synthesis by statins, atherogenesis, carcinogenesis and aging may follow. Superoxide dismutase and catalase are also deactivated by statin, although its mechanisms are unknown (Fig. 4).[15] Significance of glutathione peroxidase activity in erythrocytes was clearly shown in a clinical study; when patients with CHD were followed up for 5.4 years, the enzyme activity was inversely associated with CHD events and positively with event-free survival, and both relationships were linear.[16]

Thus, statins are mitochondrial toxins making all cells more or less ATP-depleted. Because most mammalian cells depend on mitochondria for their energy metabolism, statins are general cell toxins.

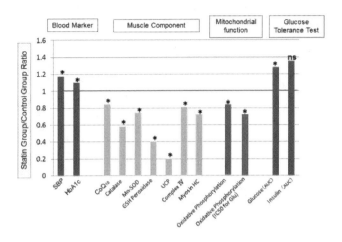

FIGURE 4 **Effects of simvastatin on skeletal muscle**

*Ten male hypercholesterolemic patients (45 ± 6 years of age) treated with simvastatin (average: 5 years) and nine controls (45 ± 4) matched for age, weight, BMI, fat percentage, and maximal oxygen uptake were compared. * P<0.05; SOD: superoxide dismutase; GSH: glutathione; UPC: uncoupling protein; HC: heavy chain; SBP: systolic blood pressure; AUC: area under curve (glucose and insulin levels were measured in a glucose tolerance test). Reproduced from figure 4 of reference #1.*

2. Statins cause coronary artery calcification

Coronary artery calcification (CAC) associated with statins has been detected by various methods over the past decade. Interestingly, this type of calcification is believed by some statin proponents as beneficial, since calcified plaque is presumably more stable and less likely to rupture.

2-1. Statins inhibit vitamin K2 synthesis

Vitamin K1 (VK1) rich in vegetable oils, contains one double bond at its phytyl side chain (Fig. 5). VK1 is metabolized to VK3 through cleavage of the side chain. VK3 is then converted to VK2 (a. k. a. menaquinone-4) by prenyltransferase with geranylgeranyl pyrophosphate. Statins inhibit conversion of VK3 to VK2 by shortening the supply of isoprenyl intermediates. In addition, lipophilic statins inhibit prenyltransferase activity,[17] the last step of the conversion. Actually, addition of lipophilic simvastatin (2.5 μM) to the incubation system containing human vascular smooth muscle cells with VK3 (2.0 μM) decreased VK2 production to 18% of the control value without statin. Thus, statins inhibit VK2 production at two different points.[18]

γ-Carboxylation of glutamyl residues is an important conversion for proper functioning of coagulation factors and osteocalcin. In this conversion VK2 acts as the vital cofactor. In bone, blood vessel, lung, heart and kidney VK2 again works as the cofactor in carboxylation of matrix gla protein. Only in the γ-carboxylated form gla protein can hold calcium and protect blood vessels from calcification. Chronic use of warfarin, which inhibits reactivation of VKs, is known to accelerate artery calcification,[19] a good marker of coronary events (see below). Similarly, statins cause artery calcification by reducing VK2 availability as shown below.

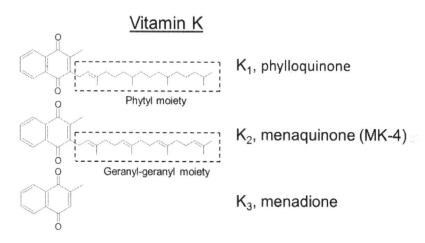

Vitamin K

K$_1$, phylloquinone

Phytyl moiety

K$_2$, menaquinone (MK-4)

Geranyl-geranyl moiety

K$_3$, menadione

FIGURE 5 Chemical structures of vitamin K

Vitamin K2 is the most important vitamin K.

2-2. Implications of coronary calcification and coronary events

In a cross-sectional study by Reaven *et al.*,[20] 309 veterans aged > 40 with type 2 diabetes with or without stable cardiovascular disease were investigated for coronary artery and abdominal aorta calcification. They noticed a strikingly higher incidence of peripheral and coronary artery disease, and all combined cardiovascular disease of 5- to 13-fold with increasing quintiles of CAC; and 2- to 3-fold with increasing abdominal aorta calcification. These associations did not disappear even after adjustment for standard cardiovascular risk factors and lifestyle parameters.

Detrano *et al.*[21] investigated CAC scores by CT and traditional coronary risk factors in 6722 men and women of four races, and followed them for a median of 3.8 years. They found that the adjusted risk of a major coronary event (myocardial infarction and coronary death) was enhanced 7.73 times when coronary calcium scores were between 101 and 300, and 9.67 times in case of 301 and over, compared with those with no calcification. They concluded that coronary calcium scores provide predictive information of CHD beyond that provided by traditional risk factors.

2-3. Coronary artery calcification by statins in cross-sectional and clinical studies

In a cross-sectional study by Nakazato *et al.*[22] 2413 patients on statins and 4260 patients not on statins were investigated for the relationship between statin administration and plaque composition types: non-calcified (NCP), mixed (MP), or calcified (CP). Their mean age was 59 ± 11 years of age. Compared with non-statin users, increased presence of MP (OR 1.46; 95% CI, 1.27-1.68), and of CP (OR 1.54; 95% CI 1.36-1.74), but not of NCP (OR 1.11; 95% CI 0.96-1.29) was observed with statin use in multivariable analyses. Also increasing numbers of coronary segments with MP (OR 1.52, 95% CI 1.34-1.73) and CP (OR 1.52, 95% CI 1.36-1.70) were associated with statin use.

In the Veterans Affairs Diabetes Trial (VADT)[23] 197 severely atherosclerotic participants with type 2 diabetes mellitus (duration,12 ± 8 years; 61±9 years) were studied. CAC and aortic artery calcification (AAC) were followed up for an average duration of 4.6 years. Volumetric scores of calcifications were assessed by computed tomography. Use of statins was encouraged in this trial because one of the interventional points of the VADT was "optimizing" lipid levels.

At baseline, 61% (n = 121) of participants were administered statins. During the study, 82% (n = 161) reported frequent statin use with a median use of 95%. Eighteen percent (n = 36) reported less-frequent statin use in (a median use of 14%).[23] Progression of CAC was significantly higher in more frequent statin users than in less frequent users with adjustment for baseline CAC and other confounders (mean ± SE, 8.2 ± 0.5 mm³ vs. 4.2 ± 1.1 mm³; p < 0.01). In those not receiving statins at the baseline examination, progressions of both CAC and AAC were significantly higher in those who subsequently reported frequent statin use than less frequent users, with adjustment for age and baseline calcium, (CAC progression, 7.9 ± 0.8 vs. 3.5 ± 1.0 mm³; p<0.01; AAC progression, 11.9 ± 1.3 vs. 7.6 ± 1.6 mm³; p = 0.04).

PURI et al.[24] investigated whether statins changed coronary atheroma/calcification in patients under high-intensity statin therapy (HIST), low-intensity statin therapy (LIST), and no-statin therapy from 8 prospective randomized trials in which a coronary intravascular ultrasound technique was employed. Patients were analyzed in a post-hoc patient-level study. Percent atheroma volume was decreased in the HIST participants from baseline, and increased in both LIST and no-statin therapy participants. Coronary calcification significantly increased in each therapy group, but statin use was associated with coronary calcium index as follows: changes in coronary calcification from baseline (median [interquartile range], mm³) in high intensity-, low intensity-, and no-statin groups were 0.044 [0.0-0.12], 0.038 [0.0-0.11], and 0.020 [0.0-0.10] (significantly different from statin groups), respectively, with adjustment for baseline calcium index ranks, baseline plaque burden (%), change in plaque burden (%), and clinical trial. Numerous limitations of the methodology of Puri et al.'s investigation are listed in comments by Shaw et al.,[25] which include less reliable intravascular ultrasound than coronary CT angiography. Nonetheless, the association of enhanced CAC by statin use was again detected. Interestingly, CAC by statin is sometimes discussed as a good prognostic sign for coronary artery events.[25] Puri et al.[24] also reached a similar conclusion. If CAC without statin is bad, and CAC with statin is good, the argument for statin seems opportunistic.

Schlieper et al.[26] indicated that patients with lower matrix Gla protein levels had an elevated cardiovascular and all-cause mortality of patients with end-stage kidney disease (ESRD). In another study,

Chen *et al.*[18] determined CAC Agatston score, interleukin-6, high-sensitivity C-reactive protein, tumor necrosis factor, in 240 patients with ESRD taking statins, and analyzed their associations with all-cause mortality. They found age, gender, diabetes and statin use were independent predictors of 1-SD higher CAC scores. Statin therapy was found to be associated with enhanced progression of CAC through repeated CAC imaging in 35 patients. The relationship between CAC and all-cause mortality was significant even after adjustment for age, gender, diabetes, CVD, use of statins, protein-energy wasting and inflammation-related factors (Fig. 6).

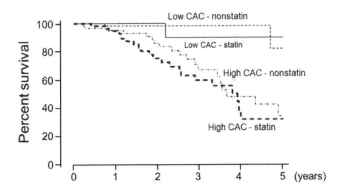

FIGURE 6 Patients with low CAC live longer

ESRD patients were divided by CAC Agatston scores and by statin use. All-cause mortality is shown by Kaplan–Meier survival curves. Low CAC: ≤ 100 Agatston Units; High CAC: > 100. Statin use did not indicate survival superiority compared to controls. (See text.) Reproduced from figure 1 (b) of the reference 25.

In this section we discussed the adverse effects of reducing VK2 by statins. These effects lead to CAC-containing coronary atherosclerosis and may induce coronary heart disease.

3. Conclusion

By reducing prenyl intermediates (isopentenyl PP, geranyl PP, farnesyl PP etc.), statins reduce heme A, CoQ10, VK2, isoprenyl tRNA etc.

158

Mitochondrial disorder by reduction of heme A and CoQ10 contents can result in malfunction of ATP-rich organs like the heart. In fact, it is highly likely that HF has been increasing in Japan. Statins inhibit VK2 production at two steps. VK2 reduction leads to serious problems like CAC, a reliable, independent predictor of all-cause mortality. Statins are poisonous to weak patients – especially to those with infection, malnutrition or little life expectancy, those with near failure of any organs, and elderly people. In addition, it is important to emphasize that retrospective epidemiological studies can only demonstrate associations, not causation.

Harumi Okuyama* PhD, Tomohito Hamazaki** MD, PhD, Paul J. Rosch*** MD

* Professor Emeritus, Nagoya City University, and Institute for Consumer Science and Human Life, Kinjo Gakuin University, 2-1723 Omori, Moriyama, Nagoya 463-8521, Japan

**Emeritus Professor, Toyama University, and Toyama Jonan Onsen Daini Hospital, 1-13-6 Taromaru-Nishimachi, Toyama-City, Toyama 939-8271, Japan

*** Clinical Professor of Medicine and Psychiatry, New York Medical College, Valhalla, NY, USA and Chairman, The American Institute of Stress, Weatherford TX, USA

Corresponding author: Tomohito Hamazaki,
hamazakit2016@gmail.com

References

1. Okuyama H, Langsjoen PH, Hamazaki T, *et al.* Statins stimulate atherosclerosis and heart failure: pharmacological mechanisms. Expert Rev Clin Pharmacol 2015;8:189-99.

2. Turunen M, Olsson J, Dallner G. Metabolism and function of coenzyme Q. Biochim Biophys Acta 2004;1660:171-99.

3. Qu H, Meng YY, Chai H, *et al.* The effect of statin treatment on circulating coenzyme Q10 concentrations: an updated meta-analysis of randomized controlled trials. Eur J Med Res 2018;23:57.

4. Qu H, Guo M, Chai H, Wang WT, Gao ZY, Shi DZ. Effects of Coenzyme Q10 on Statin-Induced Myopathy: An Updated Meta-Analysis of Randomized Controlled Trials. J Am Heart Assoc 2018;7:e009835.

5. Kjekshus J, Apetrei E, Barrios V, et al. Rosuvastatin in older patients with systolic heart failure. N Engl J Med 2007;357:2248-61.

6. Tavazzi L, Maggioni AP, Marchioli R, et al. Effect of rosuvastatin in patients with chronic heart failure (the GISSI-HF trial): a randomised, double-blind, placebo-controlled trial. Lancet 2008;372:1231-9.

7. Chin KL, Wolfe R, Reid CM, et al. Does Statin Benefits Patients with Heart Failure Undergoing Percutaneous Coronary Intervention? Findings from the Melbourne Interventional Group Registry. Cardiovasc Drugs Ther 2018;32:57-64.

8. Fröhlich H, Raman N, Tager T, et al. Statins attenuate but do not eliminate the reverse epidemiology of total serum cholesterol in patients with non-ischemic chronic heart failure. Int J Cardiol 2017;238:97-104.

9. Preiss D, Campbell RT, Murray HM, et al. The effect of statin therapy on heart failure events: a collaborative meta-analysis of unpublished data from major randomized trials. Eur Heart J 2015;36:1536-46.

10. Kutner JS, Blatchford PJ, Taylor DH, Jr., et al. Safety and benefit of discontinuing statin therapy in the setting of advanced, life-limiting illness: a randomized clinical trial. JAMA Intern Med 2015;175:691-700.

11. National Heart L, Blood Institute ACTN, Truwit JD, et al. Rosuvastatin for sepsis-associated acute respiratory distress syndrome. N Engl J Med 2014;370:2191-200.

12. Papazian L, Roch A, Charles PE, et al. Effect of statin therapy on mortality in patients with ventilator-associated pneumonia: a randomized clinical trial. JAMA 2013;310:1692-700.

13. Hamazaki T, Okuyama H, Ogushi Y, Hama R. Towards a Paradigm Shift in Cholesterol Treatment. A Re-examination of the Cholesterol Issue in Japan. Ann Nutr Metab 2015;66 Suppl 4:1-116.

14. Beck MA, Levander OA, Handy J. Selenium deficiency and viral infection. J Nutr 2003;133:1463S-7S.

15. Larsen S, Stride N, Hey-Mogensen M, et al. Simvastatin effects on skeletal muscle: relation to decreased mitochondrial function and glucose intolerance. J Am Coll Cardiol 2013;61:44-53.

16. Blankenberg S, Rupprecht HJ, Bickel C, et al. Glutathione peroxidase 1 activity and cardiovascular events in patients with coronary artery disease. N Engl J Med 2003;349:1605-13.

17. Hirota Y, Nakagawa K, Sawada N, et al. Functional characterization of the vitamin K2 biosynthetic enzyme UBIAD1. PLoS One 2015;10:e0125737.

18. Chen Z, Qureshi AR, Parini P, et al. Does statins promote vascular calcification in chronic kidney disease? Eur J Clin Invest 2017;47:137-48.

19. Price PA, Faus SA, Williamson MK. Warfarin causes rapid calcification of the elastic lamellae in rat arteries and heart valves. Arterioscler Thromb Vasc Biol 1998;18:1400-7.

20. Reaven PD, Sacks J, Investigators for the V. Coronary artery and abdominal aortic calcification are associated with cardiovascular disease in type 2 diabetes. Diabetologia 2005;48:379-85.

21. Detrano R, Guerci AD, Carr JJ, et al. Coronary calcium as a predictor of coronary events in four racial or ethnic groups. N Engl J Med 2008;358:1336-45.

22. Nakazato R, Gransar H, Berman DS, et al. Statins use and coronary artery plaque composition: results from the International Multicenter CONFIRM Registry. Atherosclerosis 2012;225:148-53.

23. Saremi A, Bahn G, Reaven PD, VADT Investigators. Progression of vascular calcification is increased with statin use in the Veterans Affairs Diabetes Trial (VADT). Diabetes Care 2012;35:2390-2.

24. Puri R, Nicholls SJ, Shao M, et al. Impact of statins on serial coronary calcification during atheroma progression and regression. J Am Coll Cardiol 2015;65:1273-82.

25. Shaw LJ, Narula J, Chandrashekhar Y. The never-ending story on coronary calcium: is it predictive, punitive, or protective? J Am Coll Cardiol 2015;65:1283-5.

26. Schlieper G, Westenfeld R, Kruger T, et al. Circulating nonphosphorylated carboxylated matrix gla protein predicts survival in ESRD. J Am Soc Nephrol 2011;22:387-95.

Cholesterol and Deaths –
The World Relationship

Zoë Harcombe, PhD

In November 2010, with a couple of hours to spare before a Wales vs. Australia rugby match, I decided to review some of the World Health Organisation (WHO) data. The WHO has extensive data from almost 200 countries on more health measures than you could imagine. I decided to look at average cholesterol levels and deaths – both from cardiovascular disease (CVD) and from all-causes.[1]

It didn't take that long – I was sat down in time for the rugby. The data have not been updated since I did this. I went to the statistics area of the WHO web site.[2] At the time, there were data for cholesterol under risk factors (which was rather judgemental to start with). I then looked under: Global burden of disease (mortality); All causes; Non communicable diseases and then Cardiovascular disease (shortened to CVD). CVD deaths included ischemic heart disease and cerebrovascular disease – that means fatal heart attacks and fatal strokes to us. I found the most recent year that provided both sets of data – so that cholesterol and deaths could be compared for the same time period. That turned out to be 2002. I downloaded their user-friendly spreadsheet data (CSV) – cut and paste it into an excel file and then tried to remember how to do scatter diagrams.

The WHO data was split into men and women. I first did the scatter diagrams for average (mean) cholesterol levels and CVD deaths for men and then women. Then I ran the Pearson correlation coefficient on these numbers. This gives us the term called "r". "r" tells us if there is a relationship: an r score of 0 would indicate no relationship; an r score of 1 would indicate a perfect relationship. A negative r score is called an inverse relationship e.g. the price of concert tickets is likely to be inversely related to the number of concert tickets bought – fewer tickets being bought at higher prices.

The "r" score for men revealed that there was a small relationship of 0.13 – however this relationship was inverse. The diagram and correlation showed that higher cholesterol levels were associated with lower CVD deaths and lower cholesterol levels were associated with higher CVD deaths. In women, the relationship was stronger – to the point of being meaningful. The r score was 0.52 – but, again, inverse. For women, higher cholesterol levels were quite significantly associated with lower CVD deaths and lower cholesterol levels were quite significantly associated with higher CVD deaths. Please note that I have added r squared on the graphs below. The r squared tells us the strength of any relationship we have observed.

Excel automatically adds the trend line. In all four graphs that follow, the trend lines go down from left to right. Immediately one wonders how we ever got away with telling people that cholesterol causes heart disease. High cholesterol is associated with lower heart disease and vice versa – for all the data available in the world.

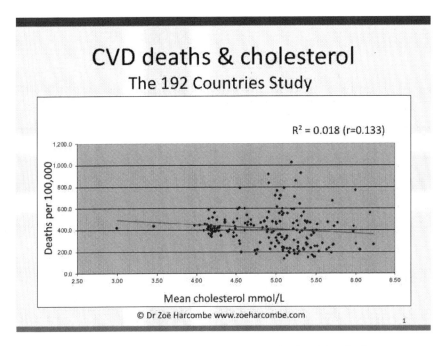

FIGURE 1 **WHO data for CVD death rates & cholesterol (males)**

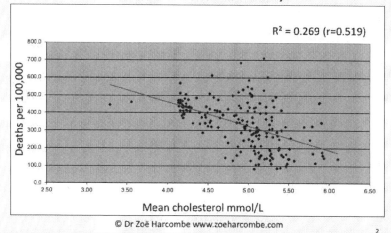

FIGURE 2 WHO data for CVD death rates & cholesterol (females)

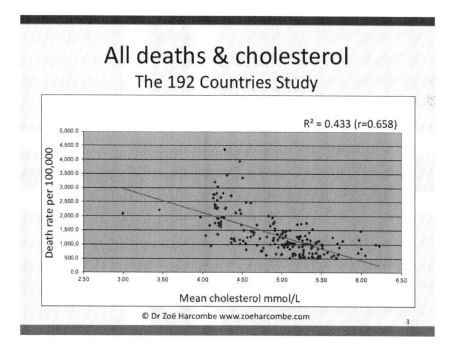

FIGURE 3 WHO data for all deaths & cholesterol (males)

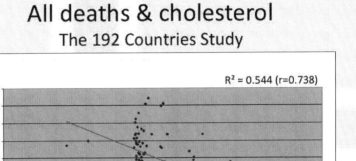

© Dr Zoë Harcombe www.zoeharcombe.com

FIGURE 4 WHO data for all deaths & cholesterol (females)

It got worse. I then kept the cholesterol information and changed the death rates to total deaths – all deaths from any cause – cancer, heart disease, diabetes, strokes – all deaths. You can see the diagrams for men and women again below. This time there is a significant relationship for both men and women: r=0.66 for men and r=0.74 for women – again inverse. There is a significant association between higher cholesterol levels and lower deaths and lower cholesterol levels and higher deaths for men and an even more significant relationship for women.

These graphs are important. I've shown these graphs to academics at professor level, with whom I've been having debates, as I want to see what the view is from people who wholly believe the fat/cholesterol/heart/death hypothesis. It is most useful to know what the resistance arguments will be before starting to invite the resistance. The two arguments I got back were:

1) "Ah yes – but this is only an association."

Ah yes – but:

1. we changed global dietary advice back in 1977-1983 on the back of an *association* in seven (carefully hand-picked) countries that became to be considered as causation even when the association was far from established;[3] and

2. it is an association that's the opposite to the one that the world currently holds true; and

3. that's what epidemiology is supposed to be about – establish an association and then investigate if there could be any causation or useful learnings. So – go out with a new belief – that high cholesterol is associated with low deaths and then see what dietary advice emerges.

(Please note that we must not make the same mistake and leap from these observed associations to causation – we can no more say that high cholesterol causes low deaths than others could claim that high cholesterol causes high deaths).

2) "But that's total cholesterol – the key thing is the ratio of good to bad cholesterol."

That is what people thought back in 2010. The obvious flaw in this argument is that there is no such thing as good or bad cholesterol. The chemical formula for cholesterol is $C_{27}H_{46}O$. There is no good version or bad version. HDL is ignorantly referred to as 'good' cholesterol and LDL is ignorantly referred to as 'bad' cholesterol. They are not even cholesterol, let alone good cholesterol or bad cholesterol. They are lipoproteins and lipoproteins *carry* cholesterol (they also carry triglyceride, phospholipids and protein).

People would now likely say "But that's total cholesterol – the key thing is LDL-cholesterol" because the cholesterol hypothesis mutates constantly. Yes, but LDL-cholesterol is the major part of total cholesterol and so if the relationship with total cholesterol is inverse, then the relationship with LDL-cholesterol is likely to be inverse.

Back to – these graphs are important. Our global dietary advice was changed in 1977 in the US and 1983 in the UK largely as a result of a biased study of seven handpicked countries.[4] Had the data been available for the 192 countries we can analyse now, or had Keys even considered all the data that was available to him at the time (for France etc), our conclusion may have been that we need to protect cholesterol levels in the body. We may have realised that the last thing we should be trying to do is lowering cholesterol – unless we're trying to lower life expectancy for some reason.

Zoë Harcombe, PhD

Independent Researcher
www.zoeharcombe.com

References

1. http://www.zoeharcombe.com/2010/11/cholesterol-heart-disease-there-is -a-relationship-but-its-not-what-you-think/

2. https://www.who.int/gho/en/

3. Keys *et al.*, "The Seven Countries Study: Volumes I-XX", Circulation, (April 1970).

4. Keys *et al.*, "The Seven Countries Study: Volumes I-XX", Circulation, (April 1970).

Do Statins Cause or Prevent Cancer?

Paul J. Rosch MD

If you do an internet or PubMed search on statins and cancer, you will find support for a causal link between statins and various cancers, just as many or more claiming that statins prevent and should be used to treat these same malignancies, with the vast majority maintaining that they have no effect at all. How can these discrepancies be explained? The lack of an effect is easy to understand, since the average statin trial only lasts 3.3 years, and it can take decades for carcinogens like smoking and asbestos to cause symptoms or signs of lung cancer. In addition, there are other factors that can accelerate or hinder this. For example, smokers who are exposed to asbestos have a risk of developing lung cancer that is greater than the individual risks from asbestos and smoking combined, and quitting smoking reduces risk of lung cancer in asbestos-exposed workers. Explaining, and especially proving that statins cause or prevent cancer is much more difficult, since it requires delineating plausible mechanisms of action, as well as long-term prospective studies, rather than metanalyses of observational studies.

How Could Statins Cause Cancer?

Statins block the production of squalene, an intermediate metabolite in the synthesis of choline that has been shown to have anti-cancer activities and is used as adjunctive therapy in treating cancer. The reduced rates of breast and prostate cancer associated with olive oil consumption are believed to be due to its high squalene content. Statins also block the production of Coenzyme Q10 (ubiquinol), a powerful antioxidant that has been found to have anticancer effects in several studies. CoQ10 production declines with aging and low levels have also been found in myeloma, lymphoma and breast cancer.

169

Although usually prescribed for cardiovascular indications, CoQ10 is also a popular adjuvant therapy for various malignancies.

Statins can stimulate the growth of new blood vessels that malignancies require to proliferate. Statins also interfere with the synthesis of bile acids, and decreased bile production can impair and slow digestive functions. The resultant increased transit time in the gut could contribute to bowel cancers. In addition, LDL " bad" cholesterol is actually "good", because it binds to and inactivates microorganisms and their toxic products. Healthy individuals with low LDL have a greater risk of both infectious diseases and cancer, which is not surprising, since microbes are thought to cause up to 20% of all cancers. Recent advances in DNA and RNA analysis suggest that as many as 40% of cancers may be due to viruses, many of which had not been previously detected.

The Immune System. Cancer and Regulatory T Cells (Tregs)

The immune system is composed of various white cells, Including lymphocytes, neutrophils, monocytes and macrophages. There are three types of lymphocytes, B cells (derived from bone marrow), T cells (made in the thymus) and NK (natural killer cells) found in the spleen and peripheral blood. These all have different functions. B cells are responsible for the "memory" functions of the immune system, since they can recognize pathogens and cancer cells and activate the immune system to eradicate them. A subset of T cells, helper T cells, assist in this response. The immune system also includes: the tonsils, which make antibodies, lymph nodes and vessels that filter and trap pathogens and activate antibodies, and the spleen, which removes old or damaged blood cells and platelets and helps destroy bacteria and other foreign substances.

When B and T helper cell activity become excessive, as in cancer, the production of Tregs (regulatory T cells) is stimulated. These were originally labeled suppressor cells, since they suppress the activity of the immune system by blocking antigen production and also suppress helper T cells secreting inhibitory cytokines and removing helper T cells by increasing their rate of apoptosis. A huge increase in Treg infiltration has been found in most solid cancers and some leukaemias. A high number of Tregs is also often associated with poorer prognosis and survival rates.

As a result, there have been increased attempts to find ways to reduce the number of Tregs in cancer patients that could improve the results of chemotherapy, radiation, and surgery. It is also important to avoid drugs like statins, which increase Tregs, as well as susceptibility to cancers, especially those that may be due to bacteria or viruses.

Several statin trials have reported an increase in various malignancies and statins are carcinogenic in experimental animals at doses that approximate those used clinically. However, it is not clear if this is due to a specific drug effect or lipid lowering, since low cholesterol *per se* is associated with an increase in cancer. The degree of LDL lowering may also correlate with greater cancer risk. Cancer is most apt to occur in the elderly who are already immunosuppressed, and in the PROSPER study, the incidence of cancer incidence was significantly higher in those 75 and older on pravastatin. The 6-year LIPID study also found a marked increase of cancer in 65 to 75 year-olds randomized to pravastatin. In the TNT study, there were more deaths in those on 80 mg of atorvastin than in controls taking 10 mg, and most deaths were due to cancer. Statins can also interfere with cancer therapy by promoting progression of tumor growth requiring radical cystectomy during BCG treatment of bladder cancer. All of the above could be attributed to a statin induced increase in Tregs.

Low Cholesterol, Low LDL and Increased Risk of Infections

Low cholesterol also increases susceptibility to various infections. In one study of more than 100,000 healthy people followed for 15 years, those who had low cholesterol at the start had significantly more hospital admissions for influenza or pneumonia, but not for chronic obstructive pulmonary disease or asthma. A review of over 68,000 deaths from 19 large studies, similarly found that low cholesterol increased risk of dying from gastrointestinal and respiratory diseases, most of which were due to infections. Young unmarried males with a history of STD are at increased risk for HIV. In one study that followed such individuals for 7-8 years, those with low cholesterol at the start of the study were twice as likely to test positive for HIV than those with high cholesterol, even after excluding those testing positive in the first four years. The MRFIT study, which screened 300,000 young and middle-aged men, found that those whose cholesterol was lower than 160 after 1-6 years were 4 times more likely to have died from AIDS, than controls with a cholesterol over 240.

Low LDL is particularly dangerous, because it binds to and inactivates toxins produced by gram negative infections as well as Staphylococcus aureus a-toxin, which is produced by most pathogenic staphylococcus strains. Official guidelines to lower LDL to less than 70 have raised safety concerns. To elucidate this, 203 hospitalized patients were divided into two groups: 79 with LDL < 70 mg/dl and 124 with LDL >70 mg/dl. There was a significant increase in fever and sepsis due to infections in the low LDL group, and each 1 mg/dl increase in LDL was associated with a 2.5% relative decrease in fever and sepsis. Low LDL was also associated with an increase in hematological cancers. In addition to bacteria, LDL provides protection from viral infections such as toga viruses that cause rubella and rhabdoviruses responsible for rabies and some types of encephalitis. As noted previously, advances in DNA and RNA research suggest that as many as 40% of cancers may be due to viruses, many of which had not been previously detected.

Over 100 years ago, Peyton Rous showed that cancer could be induced in healthy chickens by injecting them with a highly filtered bacteria-free extract from a malignancy in a sick chicken. Since then, viruses that cause infectious diseases in humans have also been found to also be associated with a variety of different malignancies, such as:

Virus	Disease	Malignancy
Epstein-Barr	Infectious Mononucleosis	Burkitt's lymphoma, Hodgkin's Disease
Hepatitis B	Hepatitis, Cirrhosis	Hepatocellular Carcinoma
Papilloma	Genital Infections	Cervical, Head and Neck Cancer
Hepatitis C	Hepatitis, Cirrhosis	Hepatocellular Carcinoma, lymphoma
Herpes	Kaposi (KSHV/HHV8)	Kaposi's Sarcoma, Lymphoma
T-Lymphotropic Virus-1 (HTLV-1)	Myelopathy/Tropical Spastic Paraparesis	Adult T-Cell Leukaemia
	Merkel Cell Polyoma Virus (MCV)	Merkel Cell Carcinoma

It is likely that others will be added to this list.

More Support for A Statin-Cancer Connection

The 1996 rodent studies showed that all statins that were then available caused cancer. But cholesterol-lowering fibrates also caused cancer, suggesting that it was low cholesterol that was the culprit. This was supported by a Framingham report in which low cholesterol and low LDL cholesterol predicted the development of cancer by decades. Nine studies that included over 140,000 individuals have reported that cancer was inversely associated with low cholesterol measured 10-30 years earlier, even when cancers detected during the first 4 years were excluded. This also refutes "reverse causality" claims that low cholesterol and low LDL cholesterol were due to silent cancers that had not yet been diagnosed. As previously noted, most statin trials only last a few years and it can take decades for a carcinogen's effect to be detected. However, in one Japanese study in which 5 to 10 mg of simvastatin was given daily to more than 47,000 patients for 6 years, cancer mortality was 3 times higher in those whose cholesterol was < 160 mg/dL, compared to others with a higher cholesterol.

As indicated. the strongest associations between statins and increased cancer risk are seen in the elderly. In other age groups, breast and skin cancers are most likely to be detected early. In the 1996 CARE trial, 12 of 286 women in the pravastatin group but only 1 of 290 in the placebo group had breast cancer after 5 years. Since some in the treated group had a recurrence of a quiescent malignancy, patients with a history of cancer have been excluded in subsequent cancer trials. And if the results of the 4S and HPS simvastatin trials are pooled, the total number of nonmelanoma skin cancers is significantly higher in the treated groups. It has been suggested that the current epidemic of nonmelanoma skin cancer is due to the widespread use of statins. The resultant increase in Tregs that inhibit host antitumor responses may be a factor in these simvastatin skin as well as the CARE trial pravastatin breast cancers. For unknown reasons, nonmelanoma skin cancers are no longer reported in statin trials.

What About Studies Showing that Statins Prevent Cancer?

But there are many more papers claiming that statins prevent prostate, bowel and other cancers, or that they provide therapeutic benefits. Since such alleged rewards are not related to lipid lowering, they are attributed to other pleiotropic effects that allegedly reduce inflammation, tumor growth, angiogenesis and metastasis. It has also been proposed that some statins can destroy a rogue protein produced by a damaged gene that may be associated with nearly half of all human cancers. In addition, statins reduce the production of DHEA (dehydroepiandrosterone) an androgenic steroid produced by the adrenal cortex, which has been shown to increase the risk of hormone-sensitive prostate, breast and ovarian cancers, and proponents claim that statins prevent these malignancies.

However, just as low cholesterol and low LDL cholesterol increase cancer risk, high cholesterol has the opposite effect, and patients on statins may have had elevated levels for decades that protected them from cancer. It is also not unlikely that some controls had low levels that put them at increased risk. Since 1996, the exclusion of all patients with a history of cancer from statin trials makes it impossible to determine whether there might have been recurrences, which could also influence the results.

What the Public and Physicians are Likely to Read

As Mark Twain warned, *"If you don't read the newspapers you are uninformed. If you do read the newspapers you are misinformed."* The same holds true for television. The following 3 U.K. headlines are taken from one of Malcolm Kendrick's excellent blogs.

- Statins slash risk of death by cancer: They slow tumour growth by up to 50% reveal major studies.

- Experts say there is 'overwhelming' evidence that statins can treat cancer.

- Study showed they cut death rates for bone cancer patients by 55 per cent.

I can add the following from the U.S.

- Do Statins Prevent Prostate Cancer?

- Statins could reduce risk of breast cancer death by 38%.

- Statins may hold keys to future cancer treatment, researchers find.

- Statins linked to lower rates of breast cancer and mortality.

- Many of these papers are published in reputable peer reviewed journals by qualified physicians and researchers who are accurately reporting what they found from reviewing retrospective studies, so why aren't they valid? There are several reasons:

- Retrospective epidemiologic studies can only show association, not causation.

- The studies were not randomized controlled.

- Only relative risk was reported, not absolute risk or number needed to treat.

- An elevated cholesterol reduces risk of cancer and many, if not most, patients are prescribed statins for a high cholesterol that protected them from cancer for decades.

- As previously noted, statin trials are too short to detect cancer, but in one that followed patients for 6 or more years, those with low cholesterol had higher cancer mortality rates. In addition, cancer death rates increased well over 300 percent in those whose cholesterol fell the most.

In researching a topic, there is a tendency to select those items that favor your views and ignore those that are contrary. I have tried to avoid this in my attempt to explain the numerous conflicting and contradictory views about whether statins prevent or cause cancer, as well as a host of other disabling disorders.

Paul J. Rosch, MD

FACP Clinical Professor of Medicine and Psychiatry, New York Medical College, Valhalla, NY, USA and Chairman of the Board, The American Institute of Stress, Weatherford TX, USA

Suggested Reading

1. Ravnskov U, McCully KS, Rosch PJ. The statin-low cholesterol-cancer conundrum. Q J Med 2012; 105:383–388. doi:10.1093/qjmed/hcr243

2. Mascitelli L, Pezzetta F, Goldstein MR. The epidemic of nonmelanoma skin cancer and the widespread use of statins: is there a connection? Dermatoendocrinol 2010; 2:37–8.

3. Oliver MF. Cholesterol-lowering and cancer in the prevention of cardiovascular disease. QJM 2010; 103:202.

4. Sacks FM, Pfeffer MA, Moye LA, Rouleau JL, Rutherford JD, Cole TG, *et al.* Effect of pravastatin on cardiovascular events in women after myocardial infarction: the cholesterol and recurrent events (CARE) trial. N Engl J Med 1996;335:1001–9.

5. Shepherd J, Blauw GJ, Murphy MB, Bollen EL, Buckley BM, *et al.* Pravastatin in elderly individuals at risk of vascular disease (PROSPER): a randomised controlled trial. *Lancet* 2002; 360:1623–30.

6. Chang CC, Ho SC, Chiu HF, Yang CY. Statins increase the risk of prostate cancer: a population-based case-control study. Prostate 2011; 71:1818–24.

7. Ravnskov U. High cholesterol may protect against infections and atherosclerosis. QJM 2003; 96:927–34.

Part Four

Why The Cholesterol Hypothesis Prevails

Doctoring Data – Especially in Industry Sponsored Statin Trials

Malcolm Kendrick, MD

We all rely on the accurate presentation of data; we need to trust the data. This is especially true with something as important as the data from clinical studies. Because these data will be used to create clinical guidelines. These, in turn, can result in hundreds of millions of people worldwide being prescribed medications. As has happened with statins.

Unfortunately, we cannot really trust what we are told. This is what Marcia Angell has to say on the matter. She was the editor of the *New England Journal of Medicine* for many years, which is the highest impact medical journal in the world.

"It is simply no longer possible to believe much of the clinical research that is published, or to rely on the judgement of trusted physicians or authoritative medical guidelines."

This was confirmed by Richard Horton, editor of the *Lancet*, which is the second highest impact medical journal in the world:

'The case against science is straightforward: much of the scientific literature, perhaps half, may simply be untrue... science has taken a turn towards darkness."

Then we have Richard Smith who edited the *British Medical Journal* two decades:

'The poor quality of medical research is widely acknowledged, yet disturbingly the leaders of the medical profession seem only minimally concerned about the problems and make no apparent efforts to find a solution."

This is worrying, it should be very worrying indeed. But what is happening? Are researchers simply making up their findings? Is it all falsehoods? Are researchers simply lying?

The answer is that, no they are not. There is no need, data can be presented in ways that bend reality through one hundred and eighty degrees.

There was a joke from the cold war, when the US and Soviet Union were bitter enemies. The leaders agree to find the best runner they had and pit them in a race against each other, one on one, to find out if communism or capitalism could create the best athlete. (This joke can be told either way around).

The US athlete won the race. It was reported in *Pravda* (the Soviet newspaper) in the following way.

'Weak US athlete finishes second from last in International race. Soviet athlete wins glorious silver medal.'

As you can see, this is true. But you may feel it does not reflect exactly what happened. Another example comes from cancer screening, and Professor Michael Baum.

"Each year I play a game with the senior postgraduate students at a course for specialists in cancer run by the Royal College of Surgeons in England. I tell them that there are two potentially effective screening tools for prostate cancer, one of which will reduce their chances of dying from the disease by between twenty to thirty per cent, while the other will save one life after ten thousand years of screening."

"As a consumer, or as a public health official, which one would you buy into? They all vote for the first; yet the two programmes are the same, they were just packaged differently."

- One screening tool reduces the chances of dying of prostate cancer by 20-30%

- The other will save one life for every ten thousand years of prostate screening.

They are both the same, it is the same screening tool. Yet, the first figure sounds impressive, whilst the second sounds highly unimpressive. You may be wondering how this can be done. It is like a statistical magic trick. Turning a pile of rubble into the Taj Mahal.

But surely doctors understand medical statistics... This is not the case, as outlined in the paper 'Do physicians understand cancer screening statistics?'

Doctors were asked to look at a hypothetical screening test (in reality prostate cancer screening once more). They were told that the five-year survival rate from this cancer improved from 68% to 99% if men were screened. The result of this was that:

"Many of the physicians appear to have mistakenly interpreted survival screening as if it were survival in the context of a treatment trial, note the authors. After reviewing only the five-year survival rates in the scenario provided, almost half the respondents who thought that 'lives were saved' stated that there would be 300 to 310 fewer deaths per 1000 people screened."

In reality

'The actual reduction in cancer mortality demonstrated in the European Randomized Study of Screening for Prostate Cancer was about 0.4 in 1000 within 5 years.'

Of course, the strange and biased way of presenting clinical data is not confined to cancer, or cancer screening. It is widely used in reporting statin trials. Just to highlight a first example of positive spin regarding statins. The JUPITER study (using rosuvastatin) was reported as follows:

"Data from the 2008 JUPITER Trial suggest a 54 percent heart attack risk reduction and a 48 percent stroke risk reduction in people at risk for heart disease who used statins as preventive medicine. I don't think anyone doubts statins save lives."

The reality is that, in the JUPITER trial the total number of cardiovascular deaths in those receiving the placebo was twelve. The total number of cardiovascular deaths in those receiving rosuvastatin was twelve. Thus, there was no reduction in cardiovascular deaths.

Therefore, the claim that statins save lives, from cardiovascular disease, from the results of this clinical trial, cannot be made. This dissonance between the actual results of statin trials, and the way they are reported is almost universal. In fact, so many tricks are played that it is difficult to cover them all. So, I shall restrict this review to:

- Use relative risk reduction, not absolute risk reduction

- Don't report critical data

- Talk about lives 'saved'

- Use combined end points.

Use relative risk reduction, not absolute risk reduction

Here, I will use a simple example to try and highlight the difference between relative and absolute risk.

You run a clinical trial on a blood pressure lowering tablet. It lasts a year, you have one hundred people taking the tablet, and another one hundred taking a placebo. At the end of the trial:

- One person taking the blood pressure lowering tablet died

- Two people taking the placebo died.

The difference in deaths is one vs. two. This is a relative difference of fifty per cent You could therefore make the statement that the blood pressure tablet reduced deaths by fifty per cent.

On the other hand, the absolute difference is one death in a hundred vs. two deaths in a hundred. This is an absolute difference of one per cent. Therefore, you could also state that the blood pressure tablet reduced deaths by one per cent. Absolute difference.

Moving one step on. You can do a clinical trial on another blood pressure tablet; it lasts a year. However, this time you have one thousand people taking the tablet and another one thousand people taking placebo. At the end of the trail:

- One person taking the blood pressure lowering tablet died

- Two people taking the placebo died.

The difference in deaths is one vs. two. This is a relative difference of fifty per cent You could therefore, again, make the statement that the blood pressure tablet reduced deaths by fifty per cent.

On the other hand, the absolute difference is one death in a *thousand* vs. two deaths in a *thousand*. This is an absolute difference of *point one* per cent. Therefore, you could also state that the blood pressure tablet reduced deaths by *point one* per cent. Absolute difference.

As you can see the relative difference remains exactly the same, but the absolute difference is one tenth of the size. Without knowing the absolute difference, the relative difference is therefore almost meaningless.

So, for example, the data from the JUPITER trial, which suggested a 54% heart attack risk reduction. What does this mean? The answer is that it doesn't mean anything important, unless you know what the absolute risk of a heart attack was, in the population studied, in the first place. Was it one in ten, or one in fifty thousand?

Which means that, whenever you see a figure such as '*a forty per cent risk reduction*' you must recognise that this figure needs to be placed in context with the underlying absolute risk.

This can be related to the prostate cancer screening figures, where a twenty to thirty per cent reduction in deaths was a *relative* risk reduction. The absolute figure is one life saved for every ten thousand years of cancer screening.

There was a very famous, and enormously successful adverts for Lipitor (atorvastatin) used in the US which stated that "*Lipitor reduces risk of heart attack by 36%.*" It helped to drive Lipitor to become the most profitable drug in the history of the pharmaceutical industry. The absolute difference in the heart attack rate, over five years, was 1%.[1]

Don't report critical data

"Clinical researchers are obligated to present results objectively and accurately to ensure readers are not misled. In studies in which primary end points are not statistically significant, placing a spin, defined as the manipulation of language to potentially mislead readers from the likely truth of the results, can distract the reader and lead to misinterpretation and misapplication of the findings."

"This study suggests that in reports of cardiovascular RCTs with statistically nonsignificant primary outcomes, investigators often manipulate the language of

the report to detract from the neutral primary outcomes. To best apply evidence to patient care, consumers of cardiovascular research should be aware that peer review does not always preclude the use of misleading language in scientific articles."[2]

The most important primary endpoint for a preventive medication is reduction in overall mortality. That is, are more people alive at the end of a study, or not? For example, if we go back to the Lipitor advert which stated that Lipitor reduces risk of heart attack by 36%, we need to ask. What happened to overall mortality?

The answer is that there was no statistically significant difference.

It is also important to ask, what happened to cardiovascular mortality? It was not mentioned in the advert, nor in any reviews of the trial. As a general rule, if an important endpoint is not mentioned, this means that it was not affected, or was not positive. In fact, this is almost a cast iron rule of clinical studies.

So, whilst it is true that the rate of heart attacks was reduced by 36% (relative risk reduction) it is considerably more important to know what happened to CV mortality. Not all CV events are fatal. The answer, once again, is that CV mortality was unchanged.

Despite this, the interpretation/conclusion of the paper was simply stated as follows:

'The reductions in major cardiovascular events with atorvastatin are large, given the short follow-up time. These findings may have implications for future lipid-lowering guidelines."

No mention of the lack of impact of CV or overall mortality.

The silence on CV or overall mortality has extended into the newer cholesterol lowering agents, the PCSK9-Inhibitors. The FOURIER trail studied evolocumab for use in prevention of CV disease. It was reported in MEDSCAPE as follows.

"After priority review, the US Food and Drug Administration (FDA) has approved a supplemental application for evolocumab (Repatha, Amgen)....

'The study, which included more than 27,000 participants with atherosclerotic CVD and already receiving statins showed that patients who received injections of evolocumab had... 15% reduced risk for composite of MI, stroke, CV death, coronary revascularisation and unstable angina hospitalisation at 22 months (P<0.001)."

"For a key secondary end point – MI, stroke, CV death... The study showed a 20% risk reduction for the evolocumab group (p < 0.001)."[3]

A 20% reduction in MI, Stroke and CV death appears highly impressive. Taken at face value this appears to mean a 20% reduction in CVD death? However, this was not the case. The total number of CV deaths were, as follows

CV deaths in those taking placebo = **240**
CV deaths in those taking Repatha = **251**

When it comes to overall mortality, the figures were, as follows

Total death in those taking placebo = **426**
Total deaths in those taking Repatha = **444**

The reality is that more people who took the drug Repatha, died. More people also died of CVD. Yet, the drug was rapidly approved.

'This study suggests that in reports of cardiovascular RCTs with statistically nonsignificant primary outcomes, investigators often manipulate the language of the report to detract from the neutral primary outcomes."

This, the non-reporting of clinical data can be a very difficult thing to spot. When a trial states that MI, Stroke and CV death showed a 20% reduction this seems to say one thing. A very positive result for the drug.

However, what is happening here is that three endpoints are being mixed together. Non-fatal MI and strokes fell, CV deaths went up. The fall in non-fatal MI and strokes cancelled out the risk in CV death. The meaning of language is being twisted as far as possible here.

Talk about 'lives saved'

If a clinical trial does reach a positive result on overall mortality this is obviously positive, and a few statin trials have shown a statistically significant effect on overall mortality. Most have not.

However, even here, the language has to be examined carefully. For example, after the Heart Protection Study (HPS) demonstrated a reduction in overall mortality, the press release claimed that:

"If now, as a result, an extra 10 million high-risk people were to go onto statin treatment, this would save about 50,000 lives a year that is a thousand each week."[4]

"The implication here is that statins save lives, as that is the wording used. However, you need to be very careful in using such language. In medicine, no lives can be 'saved.' Everyone will die at some point. Statins cannot confer immortality."

The purpose of medicine, in preventive medicine, is primarily to keep people alive for longer, not to claim lives saved. This is well recognised in other areas of medicine. In cancer trials, for example, the outcome generally used is *'increase in median survival.'* Translated this means, how much longer have fifty per cent of people lived, who took the medication.

This is extremely important, and it is the figure that patients are most interested in. Because it translates, in layman's language, into *'how much longer will I live if I take this drug.'*

Therefore, the important question, from the HPS study, would be. How much longer would a patient live, on average, if they took a statin. If we look at the figures more closely, 1.8% more patients were alive on the statin at the end of five years.
This translates to 0.36% per year (1.8/5 = 0.36).

This, if you treat ten million people, will result in 36,000 more people alive at the end of one per year, not 50,000. This can be res-stated in the following way. If you treat three hundred people, two hundred and ninety-nine will not have their lives extended, at all. One in three hundred will benefit. That, however, is a side-issue.

The next question you need to ask is, how much longer did these 36,000 people live, on average? The answer is, around four months. Which means that, running the figures, if you treat twenty million people with a statin, for one year, 36,000 of them will live for four months longer – on average. Which translates to approximately two days of increased life expectancy.

Other people have expressed the benefits of statin in numbers needed to treat (NNT). That is, how many people do you need to give a medication to, to 'treat' or prevent, one event. In the example above, the answer would be 300. As in, you need to give a statin for five years to three hundred people to prevent one event.

The problem with this metric is that you are not 'treating' a disease – in that the person does not have a disease to be treated. Equally you cannot treat death – as everyone is going to die. Using the NNT metric, whilst it has some benefits, creates the impression that a person who has not died at the end of a clinical trial, will never die. Or that death has been prevented. Or, in the case of the HPS trial you make the claim… 'this would save about 50,000 lives a year.'

This overestimates the benefit of the medication. These lives have not been saved; lifespan has been increased. Equally, nothing has been treated, or prevented. Therefore, the NNT figure is also misleading, if somewhat less so. The outcome that is of most importance is life extension.

It has been calculated that

'The median postponement of death for primary and secondary prevention trials were 3.2 and 4.1 days, respectively."[5]

This would over an average length of time of five years. So, it can be stated that taking a statin in primary prevention will extend lifespan by 0.6 days/per year of treatment. In secondary prevention it will be 0.75 days/per year of treatment.

As with using relative risk vs. absolute risk reductions the benefits of statins can be presented and thus perceived in very different ways.

Use combined end points

This is an increasingly common technique used in various clinical trials. Instead of using mortality, or CV mortality as the primary outcome measure, a combined outcome is used.

For example, in the IMPROVE-IT study, which was a trial on Ezetimibe (non-statin cholesterol lowering agent). Participants in the trial either took a statin alone, or a statin + ezetimibe. The primary outcome measure was a combined endpoint consisting of:

- CV death

- MI

- Unstable angina requiring hospitalisation

- Coronary revascularisation

- Stroke.

This combined primary endpoint did achieve statistical significance, although only just.

As you may have noted CV death was the most important clinical component of this combined outcome measure. MI and strokes can be fatal, or non-fatal. Unstable angina can be a fairly subjective measure, and coronary revascularisation is a clinical decision – not a clinical endpoint.

Also, an MI can occur as a result of a coronary revascularisation procedure (as can strokes), so if you decide to do more revascularisation procedures you will create more MIs and strokes. In short, these endpoints are not independent of each other.

In addition, a cardiologist will know – has to be informed – if a patient is taking part in a clinical trial when they are seen. The cholesterol level will also be known, and the cardiologist will be able to establish if the patient is taking the drug or the placebo – based on their cholesterol level. So, the trial becomes effectively unblinded.

It becomes possible that a higher number of revascularisation procedures will be done on those taking the placebo, than Ezetimibe, simply because the cardiologist knows they are on the placebo. More revascularisations will lead to more MIs and strokes. So, any positive finding may be a result of investigator bias.

Leaving that to one side, we know that the IMPROVE-IT study showed a statistically significant benefit on the combined endpoint of the trial. As such it was hailed as a success. A 'game changer.'

However, if we look at the most important outcome that made up the combined endpoint it was CV death. What was the difference here?

Death from 'CV causes' simvastatin = **538**

Death from 'CV cause's simvastatin + ezetimibe = **537**

Essentially, there was no change in CV deaths. This trial was commented on by Dr Sanjay Kaul, who was not affiliated with the trial.

"He said the IMPROVE-IT trial 'technically' won on the primary end point, but he questions the clinical significance of the findings, noting the overall treatment effect was modest. He also points out that the difference in the composite end point 'was elevated to the lofty pedestal of statistical significance simply due to the large sample size. A classic, example of a disconnect between statistical and clinical importance."

"Are we to applaud and celebrate a 6% relative risk reduction in a quintuplet end point that is primarily driven by reductions in nonfatal endpoint? Asked Kaul. He added that 'It is not clear which type of MIs, spontaneous or periprocedural, [happening due to revascularisation] were reduced by treatment."

The recent trials on newer cholesterol lowering agents have all used this combined end-point strategy. Claiming significance on endpoints, such as revascularisation, which do not have any clinical significance.

Summary

I have only looked at four areas where data can be manipulated in cardiovascular trials. There are many, many, more. Hopefully it has become a little clearer how data manipulation can be used to make non-significant results seems important and highly beneficial. It is up to everyone reading clinical trials reports to be aware of this type of bias and try to work out for themselves what is being said, what has been found, and whether or not to take action.

Malcolm Kendrick, MD

General Practitioner in the UK
Independent Researcher
www.drmalcolmkendrick.org

References

1. Sever *et al.* Prevention of coronary and stroke events with atorvastatin in hypertensive patients who have average or lower-than-average cholesterol concentrations, in the Anglo-Scandinavian Cardiac Outcomes Trial-Lipid Lowering Arm (ASCOT-LLA): a multicentre randomised controlled trial. The *Lancet* (2003). https://www.ncbi.nlm.nih.gov/pubmed/12686036

2. Muhammad Shahzeb Khan *et al.* "Level and Prevalence of Spin in Published Cardiovascular Randomized Clinical Trial Reports With Statistically Nonsignificant Primary Outcomes." JAMA. May 2019. https://jamanetwork.com/journals/jamanetworkopen/fullarticle/2732330

3. Megan Brooks. FDA Approves Evolocumab (Repatha) to Prevent CV Events. December 2017. https://www.medscape.com/viewarticle/889513

4. MRC/BHF Heart Protection Study. Heart experts call for urgent action to implement new findings on cholesterol-lowering treatment. 2002. https://www.hpsinfo.org/press_release.shtml

5. Kristensen *et al.* "The effect of statins on average survival in randomised trials, an analysis of end point postponement." BMJ Open. May 2015. https://bmjopen.bmj.com/content/5/9/e007118

Why the Fallacious Cholesterol Theory Continues to Flourish

Paul J. Rosch MD

One obvious reason the flawed cholesterol hypothesis of heart disease persists, is that if you repeat anything often enough, it is perceived as the truth, regardless of how erroneous or ridiculous it is. Cholesterol proponents have repeated their claims so frequently and for so long, that the dogma has become incontrovertible. They have been able to accomplish this because of powerful vested interests that influence and, in some cases, control eminent authorities, prestigious organizations, the media and academia, as well as the FDA, Congress and other regulatory agencies that are the recipients of their lavish largesse. Drug companies have twice as many lobbyists in Washington as members of Congress, and spend over $150 million/year to influence legislation, in addition to another $20 million to support specific political campaigns. But that's just a drop in the bucket compared to the more than $19 billion a year from statins alone. Despite rules that forbid this, pharmaceutical company employees also sit on FDA panels to approve new drugs.

How The Cholesterol Cartel Deceives us

The Cholesterol Cartel refers to an extremely powerful & wealthy coalition of:

- Pharmaceutical companies that provide statins and other drugs to lower cholesterol or reduce the absorption of fats.

- Manufacturers of low-fat foods or substitutes (soy, margarine).

- Makers of non-prescription supplements (phytosterols to lower cholesterol, chitosan to bind fats and "fat burners").

- Manufacturers of testing equipment to measure cholesterol, LDL and other blood lipids.

In addition to power over regulatory agencies, medical schools (research grants, CME) the media (peer reviewed journals, print and especially direct to consumer TV ads), and organizations (American Medical Association, American Heart Association, American College of Cardiology), the cartel also influences physician prescribing habits through an army of drug representatives, illegal kickbacks, paid vacations and other perks.

The Cholesterol Cartel dupes and deceives us by

- Exaggerating benefits and minimizing or ignoring adverse side effects.

- Not releasing raw data from company sponsored trials so that conclusions can be validated by unbiased investigators.

- Statistical manipulations that emphasize relative rather than absolute risk, and doctoring data in other ways.

- Failure to cite numerous contrary publications by independent researchers in review articles and meta-analyses.

- Failure to fully disclose an author's conflicts of interest and ignoring FDA regulations for banning those with conflicts of interest from serving on Advisory Boards for approving drugs.

- Providing exorbitant funds to respected organizations and eminent authorities in return for their approval and support.

- False advertising claims for low fat foods and beverages as well as statins.

- Persecuting anyone who opposes the cartel's views.

How Lipitor Became The World's Best Selling And Most Profitable Drug By False Claims And Manipulating Statistics

Most people are unaware that, except for New Zealand, the United States is the only country that allows direct-to-consumer advertising. It is permitted in the USA because pharmaceutical companies convinced the FDA that it would help to educate the public on the availability of medications that might be appropriate for their complaints. Drug advertising to consumers is banned in all other countries since its real purpose is to increase sales as much as possible by whatever strategy proves to be the most effective, even if it means creating a new disease for a product that is not selling well. In that regard, Ivan Illich's *Medical Nemesis* introduced the concept of "medicalization", which refers to turning healthy people into patients by marketing forces that determine not only what constitutes a disease but also how it should be treated. This growing trend is facilitated by deceptive direct advertising to consumers, especially on TV.

Statin manufacturers and low cholesterol proponents are adept at providing fake news and massaging data to achieve their goals. Some drug promotions are not only deceptive, but also fraudulent. Pfizer's TV Lipitor ads featured Dr Robert Jarvik, a *"distinguished cardiologist"*. After being introduced as the *"inventor of the artificial heart"*, he turns to the camera and says, *"Just because I'm a doctor doesn't mean I don't worry about my cholesterol."* He not only takes Lipitor himself, but also prescribes it to family and friends, and recommends it for everyone because it reduces the risk of a heart attack by 36%. His two-year $1.35 million contract began in 2006 with a fraudulent commercial where he is shown sculling across a serene lake in a skilled and muscular fashion. He comes across not only as a trustworthy authority, but also a caring cardiologist who is in superb physical condition. The audience doesn't know that he is not a cardiologist, has never been licensed as a physician, nor could he legally prescribe any drug. It was doubtful that he or his family ever took Lipitor until he was hired for this publicity blitz. He did not invent the artificial heart, and the Jarvik 7 model artificial heart he is shown with never really worked and was created by someone else. Dr Jarvik has no sculling experience. The shots showing how he turned the blades perfectly to achieve minimum drag between strokes as he rowed away were of Dennis Williams, an athletic, late middle-aged accomplished rower who was selected because he was Jarvik's size and had a similar receding hairline. The close-up frames that actually showed Dr Jarvik were taken while he was in a rowing apparatus on an elevated platform to conceal that it was on dry land, with the lake in the background. Jarvik tells viewers *"I'm glad I take Lipitor as a doctor, and as a dad"* before a final shot shows his double rowing away with vigorous, muscular strokes in the distance

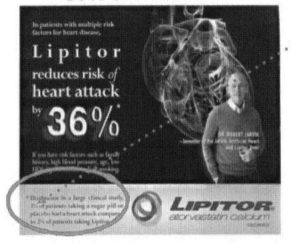

Jarvik tells viewers that *"Lipitor can lower 'bad' cholesterol by up to 60% to achieve a "36% reduction in heart attacks.*"* Few paid any attention to the asterisk after the claim that Lipitor resulted in a *"36% reduction in heart attacks*"*. It pointed to some 'small print' at the bottom of the screen explaining that there were 2 heart attacks out of 100 patients on Lipitor, compared to 3 heart attacks for controls taking a placebo. However, this 1% difference was only for those with multiple risk factors for heart disease who took Lipitor daily for over a decade. How many people would take Lipitor if they knew that its likelihood of preventing a heart attack was 1 in 100 if they took it for over 10 years? And this was only for those individuals at high risk!

The message for most was that Lipitor could reduce heart attacks in more than one out of three healthy people, regardless of their cholesterol. There was no evidence that Lipitor should be prescribed for healthy people over 65 or women of any age, except for patients with heart disease and possibly diabetes. Much of the close to $300 million Pfizer spent on Lipitor advertising from January 2006 to September 2007 was for Jarvik ads, but it was a wise investment, since thousands of patients taking other statins asked to be switched to Lipitor, which brought in billions of dollars. When Consumer Reports showed the ad to patients who had been told to lower their cholesterol, over 90% believed it was credible and accurate.

- 65% said the ad conveyed that leading doctors preferred Lipitor.

- 48% said Dr Jarvik's endorsement made them more confident about Lipitor.

- 41% said the ad conveyed that Lipitor is better than generic alternatives.

- 33% of those taking another prescription statin said they would likely ask to be changed to Lipitor.

- 29% had the definite impression that Dr Jarvik sees patients regularly.

- 20% of patients taking generic statins said they would ask to be switched to Lipitor.

Pfizer discontinued the ads in 2008 following a Congressional investigation of bogus celebrity ads and concerns that Dr Jarvik was dispensing medical advice without a license.

In 2009, Pfizer was fined $2.3 billion, for illegally marketing its painkiller, Bextra. At the time this was the largest health care fraud settlement and the largest criminal fine of any kind imposed in the United States. GlaxoSmithKline was fined $3 billion in 2012 in a health care fraud settlement. Four drug companies had previously paid over $1 billion and 13 others had paid fines ranging from $345 million to

$875 million for false advertising, which demonstrates that this is a widespread and common practice.

Personal and Professional Persecution of Cholesterol Cartel Opponents

George Mann, Professor of Medicine at Vanderbilt and a renowned nutritionist was appointed associate director of the Framingham Heart Program in 1955. His study finding no evidence that fat intake was related to heart attacks or mortality was never published, since Framingham was designed to prove the opposite, and he left. In a 1977 *New England Journal of* 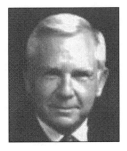 *Medicine* review entitled "Diet-Heart: End of an Era," he wrote that *"the dietary dogma was a money-maker for the food industry, a fund-raiser for the Heart Association, and busy work for thousands of fat chemists"*, and that *"to be a dissenter was to be unfunded because the peer-review system rewards conformity."*

He cited the lack of relationship between diet and cholesterol, the lack of correlation between fat consumption and death rates in the US and the disappointing cholesterol lowering trials. In 1991, Mann wanted to bring the issue before the public by organizing a conference in Washington, DC. In his invitation to prominent speakers he wrote: *"Hundreds of millions of tax dollars are wasted by the bureaucracy and the self-interested Heart Association. Segments of the food industry play the game for profits. Research on the true causes and prevention is stifled by denying funding to the 'unbelievers.' This meeting will review the data and expose the rascals."* When the cholesterol cartel found out, they sent false notices to everyone that the event was canceled. Participants backed out when they learned their funding would be cut off and the Foundation that offered to back it reneged. Mann eventually financed it himself.

Kilmer McCully, was a Harvard Professor who suggested that high homocysteine might be more important than cholesterol and could be corrected with B vitamins. Funding for research disappeared leading to the loss of his laboratory at Massachusetts General Hospital. The hospital

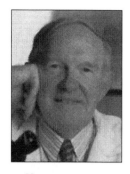
Director told him to leave and "never to come back" and his Harvard affiliation and tenure were also terminated in 1978. Although obviously well qualified for many positions that were being offered and despite the fact that he did well on numerous interviews, he was unable to find employment for two years. When he and others who had recommended him made appropriate follow-up inquiries, they ran into a stone wall of silence.

However, repeated rumors of "poison phone calls" from Harvard began to surface and it was only after a leading Boston attorney threatened a lawsuit that things suddenly changed, and he was able to resume his research at the Veterans Administration Hospital in Providence. Since then, the contribution of homocysteine to heart attacks, stroke, and accelerated atherosclerosis has been repeatedly confirmed, as well as links to other disorders, including periodontal disease and cirrhosis of the liver. He has been the recipient of numerous awards and honors, and many feel he should be considered for a Nobel Prize. Harvard has welcomed him back with open arms and even Kilmer's former critics now acknowledge he was correct.

Uffe Ravnskov received his M.D. from the University of Copenhagen in 1961 and a Ph.D. in Clinical Chemistry and Nephrology in 1973 from the University of Lund, where he was Professor of Nephrology before leaving to devote his time to private investigations. These culminated in 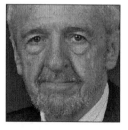 the 1997 publication of *The Cholesterol Myths: Exposing the Fallacy that Saturated Fat and Cholesterol Cause Heart Disease.* This provided a comprehensive objective analysis of the literature dealing with the role of dietary fat and blood cholesterol in coronary heart disease.

It was painstakingly referenced with numerous citations proving that a high fat diet did not cause either elevated cholesterol or coronary disease. In addition, it showed that high cholesterol actually confers protective benefits, especially in the elderly. Ravnskov's conclusions were so contrary to the prevailing dogma that he was severely berated by the bureaucracy and his book was actually burned on a Finnish TV program by cholesterol proponents. He was also severely defamed on a Dutch TV program, but critics refused to debate him on TV. They could only resort to such ad hominem personal attacks because they were unable to refute any of his claims or conclusions.

In 2003, he organized THINCS (The International Network of Cholesterol Sceptics) to inform colleagues and the general population about the benefit of saturated fat and high cholesterol and the criminal ways in which the drug industry misleads the world. It now has over 100 members including physicians, scientists and researchers, a third of whom are professors. He has written several additional books, including a revision of *The Cholesterol Myths, Fat and Cholesterol are GOOD for You!* and *Ignore the Awkward*. Additional information is available at www.THINCS.org

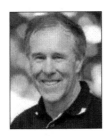 **Dr Timothy Noakes** is Emeritus Professor in the Division of Exercise Science and Sports Medicine at the University of Cape Town and a highly rated member of the National Research Foundation of South Africa. He is the author of several books on exercise and diet that support the benefits of a high-fat, low-carbohydrate diet, and maintained that high blood cholesterol was not a contributing factor to heart disease. Because of the increased popularity of this "Noakes" or "Banting" diet, he was severely criticized in the media by physicians and others with strong ties to statin and low fat food manufacturers.

In February 2014 he was reported to the Health Professions Council of South Africa for advising a mother on Twitter that she should wean her child on low-carbohydrate high-fat "real foods", rather than sugar laden cereals. A hearing was set up to investigate this allegation of unprofessional conduct but was delayed several times because of complaints that the Committee was biased and not properly constituted. It was resumed in October 2016 and a few days later, a press release stated he had been found guilty even though the trial had not been concluded. This led to more confusion and testimony from expert witnesses, including Zoë Harcombe. He was eventually cleared of all charges in June 2018 by a unanimous decision. Although completely vindicated, Noakes incurred significant legal expenses.

Dr Maryanne Demasi was a medical reporter for Australia's advertising free Channel 7 before becoming the host of Catalyst in 2006. Catalyst was the only prime time science television show in Australia, and she was awarded National Press Club of Australia prizes in 2008, 2009 and 2011 for "Excellence in Health Journalism". She produced two 2013 Catalyst episodes questioning the role of cholesterol and LDL in causing coronary heart disease and the numerous potential adverse effects of lowering cholesterol and LDL with statins.

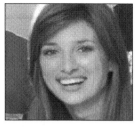

These were severely criticized by doctors and the National Heart Foundation of Australia, which published a nine-page rebuttal, which claimed that as a result of these episodes, up to 55,000 patients may have stopped taking their medication, resulting in a potential increase in deaths from heart attacks and strokes over the next five years. She disputed claims that these programs *"could cause deaths"* and explained that all the participants had reviewed their contents, and she had emphasized that patients should consult their physicians before stopping or making any changes in their medication. Nevertheless, she and 11 co-workers were terminated in 2016. Undaunted, she continued her campaign with an article in the January 2018 *British Journal of Sports Medicine* entitled "Statin wars: have we been misled about the evidence? A narrative review." It was a scathing attack on current practices that received wide support. She is now working with the Nordic Cochrane Center to promote their mutual views.

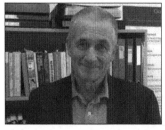

Dr Peter Gøtzsche founded the Nordic Cochrane Center over 25 years ago. Like other Cochrane Collaborative Groups around the world, it was devoted to critically evaluate medical research in an attempt to facilitate evidence-based choices about health interventions for doctors. patients and policy makers. He has repeatedly castigated Big Pharma and especially statin makers, which he views as the Medical Mafia in his books, such as his 2013 *Deadly Medicines and Organized Crime: How Big Pharma Has Corrupted Healthcare.*

It was widely acclaimed and vigorously supported by laudatory Forewords from Richard Smith, former editor-in-chief of the *British Medical Journal*, and Drummond Rennie, deputy editor of the *Journal of the American Medical Association*. He has also written numerous reviews that have criticized the lack of editorial independence of medical journals, mammography screening and the dangers of HPV vaccine. Because of these antiestablishment views, in October 2018, he was fired from the organization he founded and chaired for decades. This triggered international protests, a Go Fund Me resource for financial support, and he is establishing a new Institute for "integrity in science."

Dr Gary Fettke is an orthopaedic surgeon in Tasmania, an island state of Australia, who received a fourteen page email in 2016 from AHPRA (the Australian Health Practitioners Regulation Agency) ordering him to cease giving *"specific advice or recommendations on the subject of nutrition and how it relates to the management of diabetes or the* 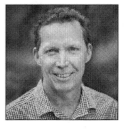 *treatment and/or prevention of cancer."* Two decades ago, he had surgery, radiation and chemotherapy for a brain tumor, and because of his interest in preventive medicine, wondered if diet played a role.

Several years later, he discovered the work of Otto Warburg, who had postulated that cancer cells can only survive if they have a constant supply of sugar. As a result, he decided that if he changed to a LCHF (Low-Carb High-Fat) diet, it might starve any remaining cancer cells. He found that he had more energy, lost some excess pounds, and that this diet also benefited type 2 diabetics, many of whom were able to stop or reduce their medication. Because of the gag order and in order to retain his license, he refrained from giving any dietary advice on his blogs, but Belinda, his wife, continued to express his views. In many ways, his situation was similar to Tim Noakes, with whom he had communicated, but Gary was judged behind closed doors, whereas Tim's was in open courtrooms. Gary's investigation was the result of an anonymous notification and throughout the process he was unaware of the peers that were judging him. It would appear that in Australia you are guilty until proven innocent, which he was. Because of numerous protests and possibly the exoneration of Tim Noakes a few months before, in September 2018, the AHPRA announced "We are pleased to report that after careful review, AHPRA has repealed its decision in its entirety, and cleared Dr Fettke of all charges. He also received the following written apology, "*I would like to take this opportunity to apologize for the errors that were made when dealing with this notification. We recognize that these errors are likely to have compounded any distress that you experienced as a result of being the subject of this investigation.*"

Almost all of the above presumed heretics have been vindicated, so is there some light at the end of the tunnel, or will fraudulent advertising and persecution of those who criticize the cholesterol hypothesis persist? Questioning entrenched dogma and distinguishing fact from fiction is hardly a new problem, and here's what some pundits have to say:

"*For every complicated problem there is a solution that is simple, direct, understandable and wrong.*"
H. L. Mencken

"*Whenever a theory appears to you as the only possible one, take this as a sign that you have neither understood the theory nor the problem which it was intended to solve.*"
Sir Karl Popper

"*All truth passes through three stages. First, it is ridiculed, Second it is violently opposed, and Third, it is accepted as self-evident.*"
Arthur Schopenhauer

"*A new scientific truth does not triumph by convincing its opponents and making them see the light, but rather because its opponents eventually die and a new generation grows up that is familiar with it*".
Max Planck

"*The great tragedy of Science – the slaying of a beautiful hypothesis by an ugly fact.*
Thomas Huxley

"The truth is rarely pure and never simple."
Oscar Wilde

"Facts do not cease to exist because they are ignored."
Aldous Huxley

"A lie can travel half-way around the world while the truth is putting on its shoes."
Mark Twain

"When I despair, I remember that all through history the way of truth and love have always won. There have been tyrants and murderers, and for a time, they can seem invincible, but in the end, they always fall. Think of it – always."
Mahatma Gandhi

"The great enemy of truth is very often not the deliberate, contrived and dishonest, but the myth, persistent, persuasive and unrealistic. Too often we hold fast to the clichés of our forebears. We subject all facts to a prefabricated set of interpretations. We enjoy the comfort of opinion without the discomfort of thought."
John F. Kennedy

"Unthinking respect for authority is the greatest enemy of truth. Learn from yesterday, live for today, hope for tomorrow. The important thing is not to stop questioning."
Albert Einstein

This topic is discussed in more detail by David Diamond's chapter in this book, as well as "Doctoring Data – Especially in Industry Sponsored Statin Trials" by Malcolm Kendrick.

Paul J. Rosch, MD

FACP Clinical Professor of Medicine and Psychiatry, New York Medical College, Valhalla, NY, USA and Chairman of the Board, The American Institute of Stress, Weatherford TX, USA

Statins – What The "Take Them In High Doses" Study Really Showed

Zoë Harcombe, PhD

The headlines on 8th December 2018 were "Stronger statins 'could save 12,000'"[1] and "Increasing statins dose and patient adherence could save more lives."[2] The article behind these headlines was published in the JAMA open network. It was entitled: "Association of a combined measure of adherence and treatment intensity with cardiovascular outcomes in patients with atherosclerosis or other cardiovascular risk factors treated with statins and/or ezetimibe."[3]

The study set out to examine how adherence and prescription intensity was associated with cardiovascular disease (CVD) events in patients recently given statins and/or ezetimibe. (Ezetimibe is a drug that decreases the absorption of cholesterol in the small intestine, which lowers blood cholesterol levels). This means that the study was trying to see if people who took their statins/ezetimibe as prescribed and if people who were on stronger doses of these drugs had fewer CVD incidents.

The funding and conflicts

The study concluded that people should take statins and take them at the highest dose. The study was funded by Amgen Europe GmbH. The conflicts of interest declared by the authors were as follows:

"Conflict of Interest Disclosures: Dr Khunti reported receiving personal fees from Amgen, AstraZeneca, Bayer, Lilly, Merck Sharp & Dohme, Novartis, Novo Nordisk, Roche, Sanofi, and Servier; reported receiving grants from AstraZeneca, Boehringer Ingelheim, Lilly, Merck Sharp & Dohme, Novartis, Novo Nordisk, Pfizer, Sanofi, and Roche; reported serving as a consultant for Novartis, Novo Nordisk, Sanofi, Lilly, AstraZeneca, Servier, Merck Sharp & Dohme, Boehringer Ingelheim, Amgen, Bayer,

203

and Abbot; and reported serving as a speaker for Novartis, Novo Nordisk, Sanofi, Lilly, AstraZeneca, Merck Sharp & Dohme, and Boehringer Ingelheim. Dr Danese reported receiving grants from Amgen. Dr Kutikova reported owning Amgen stock. Dr Catterick reported owning Amgen stock. Dr Sorio-Vilela reported owning Amgen stock. Dr Gleeson reported receiving grants from Amgen. Dr Kondapally Seshasai reported receiving personal fees from Amgen, reported serving as a consultant for Amgen, and reported receiving grants from Kowa and Sanofi. Dr Brownrigg reported receiving personal fees from Amgen and reported serving as a consultant for Amgen. Dr Ray reported receiving personal fees from lectures from Amgen, Sanofi, Regeneron, Medicines Company, Kowa, Cipla, Algorithm, Boehringer Ingelheim, Novo Nordisk, Takeda, and Astra Zeneca; reported serving as a consultant for Amgen, Sanofi, Regeneron, Medicines Company, Cerenis, Lilly, Ionis Pharma, Akcea, Esperion, and AbbVie; and reported receiving grants from Sanofi, Regeneron, Amgen, Merck Sharpe & Dohme, and Pfizer through his institution."

The study

This was a retrospective study. This means that no one was recruited into this study. The researchers simply looked at some data that were already available. The data used were from the Clinical Practice Research Datalink (CPRD) from between January 2010 and February 2016. The people reviewed for this article were *"newly treated patients"* who received their first statin and/or ezetimibe prescription between January 1st, 2010 and December 31st, 2013 and who received an additional prescription for statins and/or ezetimibe during the following year. Of the 29,797 people meeting the criteria set by the researchers: 16,701 had documented cardiovascular disease (CVD); 12,422 had type 2 diabetes without CVD and 674 had chronic kidney disease without CVD.

The rest of this article focused on the 16,701 people with CVD, as these are the people behind the headlines. eTable 3 in the supplementary file reported that 79% of these people had had a CVD event in the previous year – 55% had had an acute CVD event – and so these patients were in seriously bad shape at the baseline of the study.

Adherence was assessed annually as the proportion of days covered (PDC). Adherence was defined as taking one's meds for 80% of the days or more. Anything less than this (e.g. 79% PDC) was considered non-adherence. Treatment intensity was categorized by the reduction in LDL-cholesterol. This was also assessed annually. A 30% reduction in LDL-cholesterol was considered low intensity treatment. A 30-50% reduction in LDL-cholesterol was considered moderate intensity treatment and greater than, or equal to, a 50% reduction was considered high intensity treatment. Given that the starting LDL-cholesterol for the 16,701 people averaged just 128 mg/dL (3.3 mmol/L) and given that the starting total cholesterol averaged just 205 mg/dL (5.3 mmol/L), I cannot imagine the side effects suffered by those who managed to achieve the high intensity goal.

Flaws and issues

A major flaw with both adherence and intensity (which is what the paper is about) is that *"Measures of adherence and treatment intensity were calculated based on prescriptions during each year of follow-up and were updated annually for each patient"* (p. 3 of the paper). We know that patients sometimes don't fill prescriptions, or they fill them and don't take the drugs. This review cannot know who took what and at what intensity over the duration of the study. The paper admitted this in the discussion section: *"prescription data may not reflect the actual use by the patient"* (p. 10).

Another major flaw was the exclusion of all-cause mortality information (which was available – see "death" in the next paragraph). As Dr Malcolm Kendrick says, *"I can guarantee that you won't die from heart disease by pushing you off a cliff!"* We know from the paper that there were 3,086 events among the 16,701 people during the period of follow-up. Did people die of something other than CVD with aggressive statin medication?

The paper reported that everyone was supposed to be followed-up (and thus included in the study numbers) until: *"death; cardiovascular event of interest; last known up-to-standard CPRD record for the patient in the practice; switch to a therapy other than a statin or ezetimibe; or February 29, 2016, whichever came first"* (p. 3). eTable 6 reported the huge number of people lost from one year to the next. There were: 16,701 people in year 1; 12,824 people in year 2; 10,247 people in year 3; 6,713 people in year 4; 3,610 people in year 5 and 1,510 people in year 6. Not even 10% of the original people under review were still being assessed by year 6. Given that these people were selected from retrospective data – they weren't recruited to a study and then unfortunately lost – the 1,510 people who could be followed for 5-6 years should have been the subjects of the study.

There was a bigger issue than any of these however...

Untreated patients

The main outcome was a "composite end point" (which means lots of things added together) comprising *"cardiovascular death or hospitalization for myocardial infarction, unstable angina, ischemic stroke, heart failure, or revascularization"* (p. 3).

The results presented in the abstract of the paper focused on the 16,701 people who had confirmed CVD. The lowest risk was observed for *"adherent patients receiving a high-intensity regimen."* These well-behaved, highly-medicated patients had *"the lowest risk (HR, 0.60; 95% CI, 0.54-0.68)* **vs. patients untreated for 1 year or longer"** (my emphasis).

I immediately wondered who the untreated patients were. If the article was written looking back at 16,701 people who had been (so recently) diagnosed with CVD, surely the medical profession would have considered it unethical *not* to treat such people? Surely every one of the 16,701 people would have been offered statins and/or ezetimibe? And the untreated patients were described as *"untreated for 1 year or longer."* How could that happen?

I searched the paper to try to find out who these untreated patients were and discovered this explanation on p. 10, where the limitations of the study were being discussed. *"Because we required 1 year to estimate adherence, patients were considered to be untreated during their first year on therapy."*

So, the untreated patients were *not* a different group of patients. They were *not* a control group. They were the same 16,701 CVD patients being reviewed; only they were in their first year of treatment. That was the reference group used for comparison.[4]

Page 4 of the article reported: *"Events occurring during the first year after treatment were attributed to the lack of treatment in the year beforehand. Exposure during this period was included in the reference group (defined as untreated for ≥ 1 year)."* This means that if someone experienced an event in the first year of being on statins/ezetimibe, that event was blamed on the person *not* having been on statins/ezetimibe – i.e. being untreated – the previous year.[5] (You may like to read that twice!)

We know that the riskiest time for having a cardiovascular event is soon after having had a cardiovascular event.[6] The number of CVD events, among people recently diagnosed with CVD, would thus have been highest in the first year. This was confirmed by eTable 4 in the supplementary file. The incident rate was hugely different. There were: 136 cardiovascular events per 1,000 people in year 1; 46 events per 1,000 people in year 2; 35 events per 1,000 people in year 3; and this changed little in years 4, 5 and 6 (30 events per 1,000 people in year 6). This averaged to 72 events per 1,000 people over the duration of the review.

This study, therefore, took the year known to have the highest CVD events as the reference year. No wonder everything looked good compared to this. I'm surprised it didn't look even better. We have no idea how adherence genuinely compared with non-adherence, or how low dose genuinely compared with high dose[7] – we just know that the first year (called the untreated year) made everything else look good. Figure 2 in the paper confirms this – even non-adherence to a low dose statin was better than the reference group i.e. your chance of having an event in the first year.

Lives 'saved'

The part of the study that grabbed the headlines – 12,000 lives could be saved – came from an estimation done by the researchers. They assumed that if everyone had received the highest dose statin, and taken it religiously, there would have been 2,069 events instead of the 3,086 events that did occur. The press release reported this as follows: *"According to the team, in patients with established heart disease approximately 72 cardiovascular events were observed per 1000 patients per year. But with optimal treatment – high dose medication and high adherence – this would be expected to be reduced to 48 per year, a reduction of 12,000 cases based on the estimated 500,000 heart disease patients in the UK."*[8]

1) that's not lives saved – it's at best events avoided (and an event might be angina). More importantly 2) it's not about so-called optimal treatment – it's about getting through the first year. eFigure 3 in the supplementary file confirms that the entire difference between actual and so-called optimal treatment occurs in that first year.

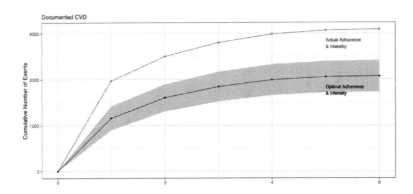

FIGURE 1 Cumulative number of cardiovascular events for actual and optimal adherence and intensity by cohort

The press release should have *said "Study confirms CVD event rate is highest soon after a CVD event."* If you get through year one without an event, the future is far rosier whether you take meds or not and at whatever dose you take or not.

Zoë Harcombe, PhD

Independent Researcher
www.zoeharcombe.com

References

1. https://www.dailymail.co.uk/health/article-6472147/More-12-000-people-needlessly-suffering-heart-attacks.html

2. https://www.eurekalert.org/pub_releases/2018-12/icl-isd120518.php

3. https://jamanetwork.com/journals/jamanetworkopen/fullarticle/2717559

4. A comment on p. 3 of the paper and some numbers in eTable 6 in the supplementary file suggested that there were some additional untreated people included in each year of follow-up. These would likely have been people who stopped collecting prescriptions for statins/ ezetimibe (probably due to side effects). The major 'untreated' group by far was the whole group in year 1 however.

5. In the supplementary file, eFigure 1 shows the timeline with everything lagged by one year. The baseline year (where adherence and intensity were zero, because the patients weren't on statins/ezetimibe) was matched with cardiovascular events in year 1. Year 1 adherence and drug intensity was matched with cardiovascular events in year 2 and so on.

6. https://www.webmd.com/heart-disease/heart-failure/news/20081104/ elevated-death-risk-after-heart-attack#1 and

S Pohjola, P Siltanen, and M Romo. "Five-year survival of 728 patients after myocardial infarction. A community study." Br Heart J. 1980. (https://www.ncbi.nlm.nih.gov/ pmc/articles/PMC482259/)

7. Not least because the supplementary file contains a lot of information but notable in its absence is the data that would show what happened within different groups of people. Incidents by group should have been presented. How many CVD events were there in the various combinations of adherence vs. non-adherent and low, moderate and high drug intensity? Then we would have been able to see the true impact of adherence and intensity.

8. https://www.imperial.ac.uk/news/189407/increasing-statins-dose-patient -adherence-could/

Statins in The Over 75s 'Save Lives'

Zoë Harcombe, PhD

Introduction

On 1st February 2019, an output from the Cholesterol Treatment Trialists' (CTT) Collaboration was published in *The Lancet*. It was entitled "Efficacy and safety of statin therapy in older people: a meta-analysis of individual participant data from 28 randomised controlled trials."[1]

It attracted much media attention on both sides of the pond. CNN reported *"After years of uncertainty, study finds statins can benefit all ages, including those over 75."*[2] The UK Times reported *"Giving statins to all older people could save 8,000 lives every year."*[3] The story took up the front page of the UK Express newspaper *"Statins really do save lives."*[4]

The CTSU

The CTSU is the Oxford Clinical Trial Service Unit. Papers from the CTSU are published by the CTT (Cholesterol Treatment Trialists) Collaboration. Following a BMJ investigation instigated by the head of the CTSU, Professor Rory Collins, it emerged that the CTSU had received more than £268 million in funding from pharmaceutical companies.[5] That was back in 2014; it can only have increased since then.

The CTSU is also the group that, despite requests from journalists and the BMJ, has refused to share information from their statin trials, so that it can be independently examined. The CTSU has also refused to share data about serious adverse events, so we have the unacceptable situation that data exist that could inform prescription practices and the holders of these data refuse to share them.

211

The lives saved claim

The claim about lives saved was remarkably consistent across the media reports:

"But scientists said up to 8,000 lives could be saved annually in the UK alone if everyone over the age of 75 received statin therapy." (The Express)

"Everyone over the age of 75 should be considered for cholesterol-lowering statins, experts have urged, after an analysis found up to 8,000 lives a year could be saved." (The Times)

"Researchers said up to 8,000 deaths a year could be prevented if GPs simply prescribed drugs costing pennies a day." (The Telegraph)[6]

"Up to 8,000 pensioners a year are needlessly dying of heart disease because they are not being given statins, leading experts warn." (The Daily Mail).[7]

The 8,000 lives saved claim came from a press conference, which was held on January 30th to launch the paper. The press conference was reported in a BMJ article, which quoted Colin Baigent as saying *"Only a third of the 5.5 million over 75s in the UK take statins and up to 8000 deaths per year could be prevented if all took them."*[8]

The problem with the 8,000 lives saved/deaths prevented claim is that it cannot be supported from evidence in the paper.

The study

The study published on 1st February was a meta-analysis of trials for which the CTSU holds data. The objective of the study was set out in the introduction: *"We aimed to do a meta-analysis of data from all large statin trials to compare the effects of statin therapy at different ages and explore the effects of statin therapy among older individuals."* The specific age of interest in the abstract of the paper and throughout the paper and in media coverage was the over 75 age group.

The paper reported that, from the available data on 186,854 people, 14,483 people were over the age of 75. Of these 14,483 people, 55% had a history of heart disease of some kind (so 45% didn't). The average total cholesterol for the over 75s was 5.1 mmol/L and the average LDL cholesterol for this group was 3.2 mmol/L. The abstract (summary) of the paper reported that *"Overall, statin therapy or a more intensive statin regimen produced a 21% (RR 0.79, 95% CI 0.77–0.81) proportional reduction in major vascular events per 1·0 mmol/L reduction in LDL cholesterol."*

There are five Figures in the paper. The only one that looked at deaths was Figure 5. It reported that the rate ratio (RR) for statins (achieving a 1 mmol/l reduction in LDL) vs. the control group in the over 75s was 0.95 (95% CI 0.83–1.07). That includes the line of no effect (1.0) and thus could have happened by chance and thus was not statistically significant. Interestingly the result for the age group 70-75 was also not statistically significant. Neither of these can be reported as a finding, therefore.

The CTT personnel even re-calculated the RRs after leaving out four trials where *"statin therapy had not been shown to be effective."* Yes – really – ponder on that for a second. Even leaving out four trials that didn't show support for statins, they still could not achieve a statistically significant result in the over 75 age group.

All the reports in the media that *"up to 8,000 lives a year could be saved"*, with reference to over 75s (or over 70s without the fudge) are false.

The evidence for cholesterol lowering in the elderly

I knew to doubt this claim as soon as I saw it because I worked on a paper published in 2016 with Dr Uffe Ravnskov as the lead author.[9] The paper was called *"Lack of an association or an inverse association between low-density-lipoprotein cholesterol and mortality in the elderly: a systematic review."* I spent several weeks doing the data extraction with Uffe and cross checking each other's tables. The conclusion was: *"High LDL-C is inversely associated with mortality in most people over 60 years."* i.e. high LDL-cholesterol is associated with lower deaths in most people over 60.

213

I also knew to doubt the *"lives saved"* claim because statin patient leaflets caution against statin use in the over 70s. Here's an extract from the Lipitor leaflet (the most prescribed statin):[10]

Warnings and precautions
Talk to your doctor, pharmacist or nurse before taking Lipitor:
- if you have severe respiratory failure

Page 1 of 6

- if you are taking or have taken in the last 7 days a medicine called fusidic acid, (a medicine for bacterial infection) orally or by injection. The combination of fusidic acid and Lipitor can lead to serious muscle problems (rhabdomyolysis)
- if you have had a previous stroke with bleeding into the brain, or have small pockets of fluid in the brain from previous strokes
- if you have kidney problems
- if you have an under-active thyroid gland (hypothyroidism)
- if you have had repeated or unexplained muscle aches or pains, a personal history or family history of muscle problems
- if you have had previous muscular problems during treatment with other lipid-lowering medicines (e.g. other '-statin' or '-fibrate' medicines)
- if you regularly drink a large amount of alcohol
- if you have a history of liver disease
- if you are older than 70 years

What about events?

Even if the death claims are lies, what about the claimed reduction in events? The newspapers reported that, *"for every 10,000 people aged 78, who take statins, but have no history of cardiovascular problems, 80 heart attacks or strokes would be prevented every year."*

This came from the press release[11] and the *Lancet* paper itself. Both identically reported *"In the primary prevention setting..."* [i.e. in individuals with no known history of vascular disease], *"Reducing those risks by a fifth with a 1.0 mmol/L LDL cholesterol reduction would prevent first major vascular events from occurring each year in 50 individuals aged 63 years and 80 individuals aged 78 years per 10,000 people treated."*

This is also false.

214

- Figure 1 reported effects on major vascular events by age. This is the Figure that gave the top level claim in the abstract of the paper as shared in "The Study" section above: *"Overall, statin therapy or a more intensive statin regimen produced a 21% (RR 0·79, 95% CI 0·77–0·81) proportional reduction in major vascular events per 1·0 mmol/L reduction in LDL cholesterol."*

- Figure 2 reported major vascular events by age and by type of trial (heart failure trials vs. dialysis trials vs. other trials).

- Figure 3 reported major vascular events by age and by type of event (coronary event, stroke etc).

- Figure 4 reported major vascular events by age and by previous vascular disease. There was no statistically significant difference between the statin group and the control group in people over 75 (or in the 70-75 age group). Benefit in those who have "no history of cardiovascular problems" cannot be claimed, therefore.

Serious Adverse Effects

Notwithstanding that no benefit can be claimed for those without previous vascular disease – and hence there will *not* be 80 fewer events per 10,000 78-year olds given statins – there will be serious adverse events in those people if they take statins.

The Number Needed to Treat (NNT) is the important measure to examine. The web site for this is www.thennt.com Frustratingly, these numbers seem to change every time I look at the page (I suspect that there is intense pressure from drug companies for these figures to be 're-visited'). Currently, the NNT numbers advise that 1 in 10 people who take statins without known heart disease will be harmed by muscle damage and 1 in 50 will be harmed by developing (type 2) diabetes.[12] So, for every 10,000 people given statins, 1,000 are likely to develop muscle damage and 200 are likely to develop (type 2) diabetes. For no benefit in heart disease.

The Daily Mail article reported Colin Baigent as having said that *"a number of misleading studies – which he branded 'fake news' – had*

created confusion over the effectiveness and side-effects of statins among doctors and patients."
The only fake news that I can find is coming from Baigent himself.

Zoë Harcombe, PhD

Independent Researcher
www.zoeharcombe.com

References

1. Cholesterol Treatment Trialists' Collaboration. "Efficacy and safety of statin therapy in older people: a meta-analysis of individual participant data from 28 randomised controlled trials." *The Lancet.* February 02, 2019. (https://www.thelancet.com/journals/lancet/article/PIIS0140-6736(18)31942-1/fulltext)

2. https://edition.cnn.com/2019/01/31/health/statins-elderly-cholesterol-study/index.html

3. https://www.thetimes.co.uk/article/giving-statins-to-all-older-people-could-save-8-000-lives-every-year-6vtt2kzll

4. https://www.express.co.uk/life-style/health/1081016/statins-save-lives-study-cholesterol-elderly

5. http://www.zoeharcombe.com/2014/08/ctsu-funding-from-drug-companies/

6. https://www.telegraph.co.uk/news/2019/01/31/75s-should-offered-statins-ageism-failing-patients/

7. https://www.dailymail.co.uk/news/article-6655239/Thousands-pensioners-dying-ageism-denies-statins-aged-75.html

8. Ingrid Torjesen. "GPs should consider offering statins to all patients aged over 75, researchers say." BMJ 2019. (https://www.bmj.com/content/364/bmj.l522.full)

9. Uffe Ravnskov *et al.* "Lack of an association or an inverse association between low-density-lipoprotein cholesterol and mortality in the elderly: a systematic review." BMJ Open. 2016. (https://bmjopen.bmj.com/content/6/6/e010401)

10. https://www.medicines.org.uk/emc/product/1059/pil

11. https://www.eurekalert.org/pub_releases/2019-01/tl-tls013019.php

12. http://www.thennt.com/nnt/statins-for-heart-disease-prevention-without-prior-heart-disease-2/

An Assessment of Biased and Deceptive Research in Diet Recommendations, Cholesterol Fears and Statin Therapy for Heart Disease Prevention

David M. Diamond, PhD

Introduction

This is a time when we have access to more information on how to improve our health than ever before. The vast amount of research findings on health and disease on the internet is both a blessing and a curse. Conflicting information abounds with regard to the foods we should eat and the medications we should take. It is understandable that confusion reigns when we are deciding how to enhance our health and increase our longevity. What is also a challenge is to determine who to trust when there is conflicting information as to what is beneficial and what is harmful. There is perhaps no greater conflict in making health-related decisions than the decision to eat animal-derived food, with its high degree of saturated fat, and whether to be concerned about having a high level of serum cholesterol.

The concerns regarding dietary choices, cholesterol and heart disease are not new, and have been a source of dispute for decades. In this chapter I have provided an evidence-based approach to address these issues. I have reviewed a largely checkered history on diet, cholesterol and heart disease, one in which high calibre research has competed with flawed and deceptive research which has been driven by personal bias and profit. I have begun with a nearly two century overview of how diet is related to obesity and heart disease. The next sections address the great challenge in understanding how serum cholesterol is related to heart disease, whether it is prudent to reduce cholesterol levels with medication, and finally, if not cholesterol, what is it that causes heart disease.

Historical Perspective on Health Concerns over the Low Carbohydrate Diet

A focal point of debates on the low carbohydrate diet (LCD) has been strong differences of opinions as to its benefits versus concerns over its adverse effects. Advocates have emphasized its effectiveness and safety in producing weight loss and in improving cardiovascular biomarkers. However, critics have warned that the LCD is a fad diet that promotes unrestricted consumption of fat, particularly saturated fat and dietary cholesterol, which has been purported to increase the risk of cardiovascular disease. I consider that the debate on the LCD has disregarded lessons learned from the long history on how different diets affect health. I will therefore provide a historical perspective on the LCD and why it became demonized as an unhealthy fad diet.

The LCD became labeled the "Atkins diet" with the publication of Robert Atkins' "revolutionary" diet book in 1972, which was almost immediately demonized as a health hazard. For example, Frederick Stare, Chair of Harvard Nutrition (1972) warned that it *"borders on malpractice ... to recommend almost unlimited amounts of bacon and eggs, heavy cream ... butter ... spareribs, roast duck and pastrami"* because of *"the well-known hazards of too much saturated fat and cholesterol"*. The critique of the Atkins diet was further endorsed by The Council on Foods and Nutrition in a scathing editorial published in JAMA in 1973, which proclaimed that the rationale for the diet is *"without scientific merit"* and further, the council expressed *"deep concern"* for *"any diet that advocates unlimited intake of saturated fats and cholesterol-rich foods."* The demonization of the LCD has continued into the 21st century with repeated warnings that the LCD, and specifically the ketogenic (very low carbohydrate) diet, increases the risk of heart disease, and even premature death.

Although the publication of Atkins' book triggered a firestorm of criticisms, readers may be surprised to learn that the LCD had been advocated without much fanfare or criticism for more than a century prior to Atkins' dietary revolution. The first recorded observation of an association between consumption of foods composed primarily of carbohydrates, i.e., baked goods and sweets, and obesity was in the book "The Physiology of Taste", published in 1825 by the French philosopher and gastronome Jean Anthelme Brillat-Savarin. His observations of

218

obese people and farm animals led him to conclude *"an anti-fat diet is based on the commonest cause of obesity ... it is only because of grains and starches that fatty congestions can occur, in man as in the animals ... a more or less rigid abstinence from everything that is starchy or floury will lead to the lessening of weight."* Brillat-Savarin specifically forbade the obese person from eating cookies, cakes, potatoes, macaroni and bread. If only for his unique style of writing and timeless message, it is worth citing one of his admonitions to the obese: *"You love soup, so have it made à la julienne, with green vegetables, cabbages, and root vegetables. I must forbid you to drink it with bread, starchy pastes and flour. Veal and poultry should be preferred. Shun everything made with flour, no matter in what form it hides".*

Decades later, the French scientist Claude Bernard discovered the capacity for the liver to store sugar in the form of glycogen, and more importantly, to generate sugar, *de novo*, from protein. Bernard's ground-breaking research inspired William Harvey, a British physician, to speculate that the liver's capacity to generate sugar from endogenous (internal) sources, meant that dietary sugar was not a required nutrient. Harvey returned to London to share this information with one of his patients, William Banting, who was suffering from obesity-related health problems. Harvey recommended that Banting restrict his consumption of sweet foods, bread and potatoes. Although Banting's diet wasn't a strict LCD, since it did include daily bread and a good bit of alcohol (and it had some quirks, such as a restriction on consuming pork and salmon), the most important feature of the diet was that it restricted food rich in carbohydrates.

In a book published by Banting in 1863 on his diet, weight reduction and improved health, he stated that he abstained as much as possible from *"bread, butter, milk, sugar, beer, and potatoes, which had been the main (and, I thought, innocent) elements of my existence".* According to Banting, he lost a pound per week over a year's time to stabilize at 152 pounds. Banting, who had been obese and ill at 60 years of age, lived with improved health into his 80's, as he remained on this diet for over two decades.

Comparable late 19th century observations of a link between consumption of foods rich in simple carbohydrates and obesity, as well as poor health, are found in an impressive compendium by Emmett Densmore, in his book entitled *The Natural Food of Man*

219

(1892). Densmore provides an extensive review of approaches by other physicians, as well as his own observations, on diet, obesity and health. He noted that people with health complaints tend to *"be greatly attached to food such as bread, puddings, pies, tarts, cakes and flour preparations in general"*, and further, that *"those seldom troubled with disease of any kind ... partake more of fresh vegetables, greens, fruits and animal food, fish, fowl, eggs ... who cared little for grain food, such as flour in its various forms"*. He blamed consumption of carbohydrates as the cause of obesity, as illustrated in his summation: *"An obese person ... may be given a diet of flesh with water, with the addition of starchless vegetables ... excluding bread, pulses and potatoes, and the patient will be gradually but surely reduced to his normal weight. ... As soon, however, as the patient returns to his usual diet of bread and potatoes he straightway begins to increase in weight ... he will gain fully (all lost weight) upon returning to a free use of bread and starchy vegetables."*

The identification of carbohydrates as the primary obesogenic agent continued into the 20th century. In the 1950s, Alfred Pennington provided a series of scholarly reviews of 150 years of research, including findings from his own research program, on the most effective dietary treatments for obese people. In one of his publications in the *New England Journal of Medicine*, Pennington described his own approach, stating that the ideal *"treatment of obesity ... is that of a diet in which carbohydrate, alone, is restricted and protein and fat are allowed ad libitum."*

A similar recommendation was provided by George Thorpe in the Chairman's address to the American Medical Association in *JAMA* in 1957. Thorpe reviewed the diet and obesity literature, concluding that *"Evidence from widely different sources ... seems to justify the use of high-protein, high-fat, low-carbohydrate diets for successful loss of excess weight."*

The recommendation to selectively target carbohydrate restriction for safe and effective weight reduction was advocated in medical textbooks in the middle of the 20th century. For example, in *The Practice of Endocrinology* (1951), Raymond Greene provided specific dietary guidelines in the treatment of the obese patient, including: *"complete restriction of bread (and everything else made of flour), cereals, potatoes, sweets, and in general, any food containing much sugar."* His text also recommended to the obese: *"You can eat as much as you like of the following foods: Meat, fish, birds, green vegetables, eggs, cheese and unsweetened fruit, except for bananas and grapes."*

In the book *Strong Medicine* (1961), Blake Donaldson admonished obese patients *"Your flour and sugar days are over for the rest of your life... No breadstuff means any kind of bread ... biscuits and crackers, ... toast ... pastry ... waffles, pancakes, all cakes ... must go out of your life, now and forever".* Indeed, one of Donaldson's assertions to a diabetic patient is as relevant now as it was in 1961: *"You are out of your mind when you take insulin in order to eat Danish pastry".* His advice to the patient was to *"eat a large amount of fresh fat meat three times a day in order to burn off your own fat",* which is contrary to contemporary warnings against red meat and saturated fat consumption, but were entirely consistent with over a century of observations on the ideal dietary treatment for obese individuals.

One final paper is noteworthy in this historical perspective on the LCD. A publication in *JAMA* by Gordon *et al.* in 1963 is unique because it advocates the use of the LCD, but the authors appear to have been unaware of the vast literature on the effectiveness of the LCD as a treatment for obesity. These authors referred to their approach as a *"unique concept in the treatment of obesity".* The rationale for their diet recommendations was based on the finding that *"low carbohydrate intake tends to minimize the storage of fat"* which was why they designed their protocol to be *"planned around the basic concept that its carbohydrate content should be low".* They reported dramatic reductions of weight in obese patients which were restricted to 50g of carbohydrates/day. As with other clinicians working with obese individuals, they reported that their subjects on the LCD lost weight without feeling hunger, and that the weight reductions were reversed once their subjects returned to a high carbohydrate diet.

This 1963 paper in *JAMA* was at a pivotal point in LCD history. It was published a century after the publication of William Banting's book on how he successfully lost weight by abstaining *"as much as possible from bread, butter, milk, sugar, beer, and potatoes",* and a decade after Pennington described the great benefits of an LCD for the obese. It is ironic that it was also in *JAMA* a decade later that The Council on Foods and Nutrition proclaimed the LCD was *"without scientific merit",* as well as Frederick Stare's condemnation of prescribing the LCD as *"bordering on malpractice".*

How is it that the LCD had been hailed as a safe and effective weight loss regimen for over a century, with descriptions of its efficacy in highly regarded medical journals, suddenly to become a form of malpractice in 1972, with continued criticism to the present day? The critique of the LCD seems surprising given that obesity is one of the greatest risk factors for heart disease and the LCD is so effective at reducing weight.

The Rise and Fall of the Diet-Heart Hypothesis

The explicit basis of the critique of the Atkins diet is the great concern that people on the LCD will consume excess saturated fat (found in a greater extent in animal fat and tropical oils), which will raise their serum cholesterol levels and therefore increase their risk of heart disease. This hypothesized linkage of dietary fat to elevated serum cholesterol to obesity and heart disease was referred to as the "Diet-Heart Hypothesis". The flawed research purportedly linking saturated fat consumption to serum cholesterol to an increased risk of atherosclerosis has been reviewed at length in numerous books, as well as in publications and will only briefly covered here.

The discovery in the first half of the 20th century of an association between a genetic basis for elevated levels of serum cholesterol (familial hypercholesterolemia; FH) and an increased incidence of heart disease led to recommendations that consumption of cholesterol, as well as serum cholesterol levels, should be reduced by diet or pharmacological treatments. Studies involving feeding of rabbits high concentrations of cholesterol produced fatty streaks (but not atherosclerosis) in their blood vessels, but there was little evidence that dietary cholesterol affected serum cholesterol in omnivores and humans. The flaws in this approach have been addressed by numerous authors who have noted that cholesterol is only found in food derived from animals, and rabbits are herbivores. The goal of finding fatty streaks was more important than sound experimental methods, since feeding meat to omnivores, such as rats and dogs, did not produce atherosclerosis.

Given the failure to relate total fat to heart disease, investigators sought to identify other dietary influences which could be associated with elevated cholesterol levels, and therefore, to explain how diet causes heart disease. The search for the influence of diet on heart disease led one investigator, Ancel Keys, to promote the diet-heart hypothesis, which, originally, was the idea that excess fat in the diet was atherogenic. Keys noticed, for example, that Americans consumed more fat in their diet, and they had higher cholesterol levels and more heart disease than people in other countries. This observation suggested to him that dietary fat causes heart disease by elevating serum cholesterol. To support his hypothesis Keys published a paper in a hospital newsletter citing evidence of a positive linear relation between the dietary fat consumed (without regard to the type of fat) and national rates of mortality from heart disease. Soon after publication of this finding, other investigators revealed that Keys had selected only a subset of all data available to him on diet and mortality. The other authors pointed out the inappropriate data selection by Keys, and more importantly, they showed that when all data were analyzed there was no relation between fat in the diet and mortality from heart disease.

Undaunted by the absence of an effect of dietary fat on heart disease, numerous investigators in the 1950s, as well as Keys, focused on the hypothesis that specific types of fat would affect serum cholesterol, thereby providing a more refined assessment of the presumed dietary lipid-heart disease linkage. Progress appeared to have been made with the finding that short-term feeding of test subjects with food high in saturated fat, such as butter, could produce an increase in serum cholesterol. Conversely, feeding the same individuals with food high in polyunsaturated fat, such as corn oil, lowered cholesterol levels. These observations led Keys to propose that corn oil could be of value in the treatment of ischemic heart disease.

The hypothesis that consumption of polyunsaturated fats with a concomitant reduction in cholesterol levels was unsupported with the outcome of the first, and only, study on the effects of corn oil treatment in men diagnosed with heart disease. Rose and co-workers in 1965 demonstrated that daily corn oil consumption produced a significant reduction in serum cholesterol levels in middle-aged men, but the trial was a failure because there were significantly more deaths and heart attacks in the experimental, compared to control, groups of subjects. The authors urged men with heart disease not to use corn oil in their diets.

In an interview with Time magazine in 1961, Ancel Keys stated as a fact that saturated fat causes heart disease, despite the complete absence of any supporting evidence for his assertions. Keys then established the Seven Countries Study, which was the largest epidemiological investigation of the relation between diet and heart disease in history. This study has been criticized by numerous investigators as flawed at multiple levels of analysis, as well as in its clear bias in interpretation. For example, had Keys included France in the study, the diet-heart hypothesis would have been dismissed because the French have a low rate of heart disease despite a diet high in saturated fat. However, the low incidence of heart disease in France has been either ignored or dismissed as the "French Paradox".

More importantly, in Keys' Seven Countries Study, as well as in other research, there was clear evidence of an association between sugar with saturated fat consumption, and the combination of the two factors was associated with heart disease. That is, people who eat the most sugar (from bread, soda and ice cream) also tend to eat the most saturated fat (from cheeseburgers), and they also have the most heart disease. Keys dismissed the correlation between sugar consumption and heart disease as irrelevant, focusing exclusively on saturated fat causing heart disease through increased serum cholesterol. There is no doubt that excess consumption of the combination of carbohydrate and saturated fat contributes to obesity and heart disease. Unfortunately, once Ancel Keys focused on saturated fat as the sole dietary cause of heart disease, findings contrary to his hypothesis were simply ignored or categorized as paradoxical.

The hypothesis that saturated fat consumption caused heart disease by increasing serum cholesterol was flawed to begin with and has not been supported by carefully conducted research. Historically, evidence from national statistics demonstrated that as the incidence of heart disease mortality in the US was increasing in the first half of the twentieth century, Americans were consuming less butter and more margarine. The irony in this finding is that the demonization of food rich in saturated fat contributed to the decline in butter consumption, which contributed to the increase in margarine consumption, which, as is well-known now, was high in artery damaging trans-fats. Therefore, if one reviews what people were eating in the first half of the twentieth century, there was if anything, an inverse association between butter consumption and heart disease incidence in the US.

In the past decade, investigators have carefully reviewed studies examining a potential relation between saturated fats and heart disease, independent of other factors, such as sugar consumption. They have reached the conclusion that there is no evidence of a direct linkage of saturated fat consumption, or dietary restriction of saturated fat, to heart disease, despite the maintenance of this view by national health organizations, such as the American Heart Association. In recent years commentaries and reviews have made this point more assertively, such as the following conclusion by Ravnskov, *et al.*, in 2014: *"There is no evidence that a lower intake of SFA can prevent CVD ... Because there is much evidence that saturated fat may even be beneficial, we urge the American Heart Association, the American Diabetes Association, and the National Institute of Clinical Excellence to consider the aforementioned evidence when updating their future guidelines."*

In the past five years there has been great progress in bringing to closure our appreciation of the kinds of food that contribute to impaired health. The latest research, spearheaded by renowned contemporary researchers, such as Richard Feinman, Zoë Harcombe, Eric Westman, Jeff Volek, Stephen Phinney and Sarah Hallberg, among many others, have confirmed what was first observed in the nineteenth century by Brillat-Savarin, Bernard, Banting and Densmore, and then in the first half of the twentieth century by Pennington, Thorpe, Greene, Donaldson, and Weston Price in his analysis of indigenous people around the world: The primary dietary component that contributes to the diseases of modern civilization is excess consumption of food that increases blood sugar (carbohydrates). A secondary component that has not received sufficient attention but is likely a major contributor to diet-related diseases, is consumption of food deep-fried in vegetable oil. The absence of these two components, sugar and food deep-fried in vegetable oil, in the diets of non-westernized and prehistoric people, explains why they enjoyed excellent health.

Failure of Pre-Statin Era Clinical Trials to Demonstrate Cardiovascular Benefits of Cholesterol Reduction

As mentioned previously, one of the first treatments for atherosclerosis in FH was based on the finding that consumption of corn oil resulted in a reduction of cholesterol levels. In 1965, Rose and co-workers tested this hypothesis with the use of corn oil consumption and a low fat, low cholesterol diet as a treatment for men at high risk of a second coronary event, compared to no treatment in the control group. Dietary treatment reduced cholesterol levels, but the trial was a failure because the incidence of coronary events and death was greater in the corn oil group compared to the placebo group.

In 1965, a trial was initiated on 10,000 middle-aged men with hypercholesterolemia who were treated with clofibrate or placebo. This study demonstrated that a reduction in cholesterol levels in the clofibrate group was associated with a small decrease in non-fatal, but not fatal, coronary events. But this trial failed, as well, because the clofibrate-treated group exhibited greater all-cause mortality than the placebo-treated hypercholesterolemic group.

In 1984, the largest cholesterol reduction RCT on record was published, in which 480,000 middle-aged men were screened to identify those at the 95th percentile of total cholesterol and an LDL-C of at least 190 mg/dl. This was the ultimate test of cholesterol lowering therapy for men at extremely high risk of dying of heart disease, based on their having such high levels of cholesterol. After 7.4 years of cholestyramine (cholesterol-lowering) treatment, there was no difference in the rate of death between the placebo-treated and cholestyramine-treated men, and only 2% of deaths of placebo-treated and 1.6% of cholestyramine-treated men were attributable to coronary heart disease, Once again, a cholesterol lowering trial in men at high risk of dying had failed to show significant benefits.

This 1984 trial, which cost the US taxpayer an estimated $150 million to accomplish, was a complete failure, based on its tacit goal to demonstrate that reduction of cholesterol would cure people of heart disease and save lives. It was a scientific success, however, in that it unequivocally demonstrated that cholesterol reduction had little overall effect on coronary events and mortality, It is remarkable that the trial director, Basil Rifkind, ignored the absence of any substantial benefit with cholesterol reduction by stating in an interview in Time magazine *"This is the evidence scientists have been waiting for. It is a turning point in cholesterol-heart-disease research."* Since the drug used in that study produced disturbing gastrointestinal disturbances, Rifkind declared *"Doctors hope that the results of the N.H.L.B.I. trial will convince pharmaceutical companies that there is a need for less expensive, more palatable drugs."* It was this trial, and Rifkind's unjustified sense of urgency for better cholesterol-lowering drugs, that ushered in the statin era.

How Statistical Deception Created the Appearance of Statins as "Miracle Drugs"

Over two decades ago, William Clifford Roberts, MD, editor of the American Journal of Cardiology, referred to statins (drugs which reduce cholesterol levels) as *"underused miracle drugs"*, which are to *"atherosclerosis what penicillin was to infectious disease"*. He announced that statins *"have the capacity to prevent (coronary) events in the first place"*. He urged physicians to *"convince patients that these miracle drugs ... are the best anti-atherosclerotic insurance they can purchase."*

What kind of findings could motivate a cardiologist and editor of a prestigious medical journal to be so enthusiastic about a drug treatment for cardiovascular disease? His praise for statins was based on findings that statins could produce dramatic reductions in the rate of coronary events, such as a 50% reduction in the rate of heart attacks.

Despite Roberts' enthusiastic praise for statin effectiveness, others were not so sanguine about their benefits. For example, early in the statin era, Thompson and Temple stated: *"The small differences favouring the drug* (statins) *have been magnified by the manner of presentation of results"*. Their objection to the praise for statins was based on what may be considered deceptive practices by statin advocates to amplify the appearance of benefits of statin treatment. Therefore, in this section I will review statistical terms which are at the forefront of the debate.

The statistical terms I will focus on are relative (RRR) and absolute (ARR) risk reduction, and the number needed to treat (NNT). To illustrate the use of these terms in clinical research, consider a 5-year trial that includes 2000 healthy, middle-aged men. The aim of the trial is to see if a statin can prevent heart disease. Half of the participants are administered the statin and the other half a placebo. In most clinical trials we find that during a period of five years about 2% of all healthy, middle-aged men experience a non-fatal heart attack. Consequently, at the end of our hypothetical trial, 2% of the placebo-treated men and 1% of the statin-treated men suffered a heart attack. Statin treatment, therefore, has been of benefit to 1% of the treated participants. Thus, the ARR, which quantifies how effective a treatment is on the population at risk, was one percentage point, and the NNT was 100. That is, when the benefit occurs to only 1% of the population, then 100 people need to be treated to benefit 1 person. Put another way, the chance of not suffering from a heart attack during the five-year period without treatment was 98% and by taking a statin every day the benefit to the population increased by 1 percentage point, to 99%. This also means that for every 100 people treated with a statin, 99 will receive no benefit.

When it comes to presenting the findings of this hypothetical trial to healthcare workers and the public, the directors of this trial do not think people would be impressed by a mere one percentage point improvement with drug treatment. Therefore, instead of using the ARR they present the benefit in terms of relative risk reduction (RRR). The RRR is a derivative of the ARR in which the arithmetic difference in disease outcomes between the placebo and treated groups is subtracted and then expressed as a ratio. In this example, the difference from 2% in the rate of heart attacks in the placebo group to 1% in the treated group, is 1%, which gets converted to a 50% reduction in rate of heart attacks. Hence, by using RRR, the directors can state that their treatment reduced the incidence of heart disease by 50%, because 1 is 50% of 2.

Expert investigators have strongly criticized this distortion of clinical study outcomes. For example, one of the strongest condemnations of the reporting of relative risk without absolute risk in medical publications was by Gigerenzer and co-workers. They wrote an editorial in the *British Medical Journal*, in which they chastised investigators who reported only relative risk in their clinical data presentation, noting that they committed the *"first 'sin' against transparent reporting."* Their indignation at this practice was expressed by their call for institutions to cancel their subscriptions to medical journals that failed to enforce transparency in how they present risk data.

It is in the context of how the selective use of relative risk measures exaggerates the appearance of the benefits of treatments that the reader can appreciate why the jubilant reception statins have received from the medical community is undeserved. Clinical trial data presented by statin advocates have been reported almost exclusively in the RRR format, which has been decried by various experts as deceptive, meaningless and leading to confusion.

One example of the use of RRR to present statin trial data is the JUPITER trial, which was published in JAMA in 2008. Rosuvastatin (Crestor) or placebo was administered to 17,802 healthy people with elevated C-reactive protein, but with no prior history of CHD or elevated cholesterol levels. The primary outcome was the occurrence of a major cardiovascular event, defined as nonfatal myocardial infarction, nonfatal stroke, hospitalization for unstable angina, arterial revascularization, or death from cardiovascular causes.

The trial was stopped after a median follow-up of only 1.9 years. The benefit of Crestor treatment, with regards to the ARR of heart attacks was minuscule. There were only 68 (0.76%) versus 31 (0.35%) heart attacks (out of 17,802 people!), in the placebo and Crestor groups, respectively. The ARR produced by Crestor was only 0.41 percentage points and an NNT of 244. This means that less than one half of one per cent of the treated population (0.41%) benefited from Crestor treatment, and 244 people needed to be treated to prevent a single fatal or non-fatal heart attack. Despite this meager effect, in the media the benefit was stated as *"more than fifty per cent avoided a fatal heart attack"*, because 0.41 is 54% of 0.76.

The public and healthcare workers were informed of a 54% reduction of heart attacks, when the actual effect in the treated population was a reduction of less than 1 percentage point. Moreover, the ARR of 0.41 percentage points was the combination of fatal and nonfatal heart attacks. There was little attention paid to the fact that *more people had died from a heart attack in the treatment group.* Even experienced researchers may have overlooked this finding because the figures were not explicitly stated in the report. One needs to subtract the number of non-fatal CHD from the number of "any myocardial infarction" to see that there were 11 fatal heart attacks in the treatment group, but only 6 in the control group.

Despite the minuscule benefits of Crestor reported in the publication, in the media the JUPITER findings were presented as impressive. In an article in Forbes Magazine, John Kastelein, a co-author of the study, proclaimed: *"It's spectacular ... We finally have strong data"* that a statin prevents a first heart attack. This triumphant declaration of victory in the war on cholesterol convinced an FDA advisory panel to recommend Crestor treatment for people with elevated C-reactive protein levels and normal levels of cholesterol.

According to a table in the JUPITER report there was no difference between the numbers of serious adverse effects between the two groups. However, in the Crestor group there were 270 new cases of diabetes, but only 216 in the control group (3% vs. 2.4%). Unlike beneficial effects, which the authors amplified in the magnitude of its appearance by using RRR, the significant effect of new onset diabetes by Crestor treatment was expressed only in the ARR form. It is notable that the increase in new onset diabetes with Crestor has been replicated reliably in other trials with different statins. The substantial increase in new onset diabetes should be a great concern to patients, but its significance has been downplayed by statin advocates.

An objective assessment of the JUPITER findings should therefore be conveyed to potential patients in the following manner: "*Your chance to avoid a heart attack during the next two years is about 99.3% without treatment, but you can increase it to about 99.7% by taking Crestor every day. However, you will not prolong your life and there is a risk you may develop diabetes, not to mention other serious adverse effects*".

Hence, in the war on cholesterol, the advocates have used as a primary weapon in their arsenal the selective presentation of relative risk values, which is recognized as deceptive because it artificially amplifies the appearance of statins to be highly effective in the treatment of cardiovascular outcomes, when in reality, the effects are quite small. The intentional exclusion of the ARR and NNT in medical reports, press releases and conference presentations by statin advocates explains why the skeptics have been critical of the accolades for statins as "wonder drugs" in the treatment of cardiovascular disease.

It is worth noting that despite the amplification of the appearance of the benefit of statin treatment, at a global level, a real reduction of coronary events and death in 1% of the population could make a substantial difference in health outcomes if statins did not have any adverse effects. However, the adverse effects are substantial, including an increased rate of cancer, cataracts, diabetes, cognitive impairment, and musculoskeletal disorders.

In summary, my goal in this section was to provide an overview of the terminology and deceptive data analyses which are routinely employed by clinical trial directors in how they convey finding to the public. I have shown that by focusing almost exclusively on the RRR format of data presentation, statin advocates have routinely provided health care providers and the public the false appearance of statin treatment to be highly effective at reducing CHD events and mortality, when the effects at the population level have been meager. Experts in the field have condemned the isolated presentation of relative risk values as deceptive. Statin advocates, by contrast, have embraced the strategy of presenting only relative risk data because highlighting the absolute risk reduction findings to practitioners and the lay public would illuminate the minuscule beneficial effects of statins on cardiovascular outcomes.

What Should Replace The Failure Of The Cholesterol Hypothesis?

One of the first studies describing premature death from coronary heart disease (CHD) in individuals with high cholesterol was by Muller in 1938. In the decades since Muller's publication, high cholesterol was so commonly associated with CHD that an elevated level of cholesterol, particularly low-density lipoprotein cholesterol (LDL), became accepted as a causal influence on the development of CHD. When Brown and Goldstein were awarded the Nobel Prize in 1985 for their work on the LDL receptor, they implicated LDL as a primary cause of CHD. Hence, the involvement of cholesterol in causing CHD appeared to be confirmed. As a consequence of LDL being perceived as inherently atherogenic, the standard of care in all contemporary guidelines for prevention of CHD has focused on reducing serum LDL levels.

However, from the earliest observations to the present, there have been findings which are inconsistent with the view that cholesterol is a causal risk factor in the development of CHD. For example, Harlan *et al.*, in 1966, and later Mundal *et al.*, in 2014, reported that individuals with familial hypercholesterolemia (FH), which have two to three times normal levels of LDL, have an overall normal rate of survival into their sixth, seventh, and even eighth decades of life. Indeed, Mundal *et al.* showed that individuals with FH from 70-79 years of age have a significantly lower rate of death than non-FH individuals with normal cholesterol.

The meager benefits of statins to reduce CVD events, despite a substantial reduction of LDL, and the long life of people with FH argue against LDL as a causal factor for CHD. However, it must be acknowledged that FH individuals do suffer from more heart attacks than the general population, but is that because they have high cholesterol or do they have another risk factor that has been largely ignored?

If not LDL as a cause of CHD, what is the alternative explanation for why people with FH, as well as the general population, are susceptible to developing CHD? The alternative hypothesis is that the primary cause of CHD is heightened platelet aggregation (excess clotting), rather than elevated LDL. My colleagues and I have reviewed the FH literature and we have found people who have a high level of clotting factors, independent of their LDL levels, have a high rate of CHD. For example, people with FH have highly sensitive platelets (cells that promote clotting) in response to stress hormones, such as adrenaline. This is an important finding which has been almost entirely overlooked by conventional (LDL-centered) analyses of CHD susceptibility. This finding means that people with FH are much more sensitive to stress-induced CHD than the general population.

Therefore, in people with FH who suffer premature CHD, the critical abnormality is one of coagulopathy (clotting-related damage), not high LDL. These findings strongly suggest that a risk factor other than high LDL, such as a highly reactive coagulation system, is the key player in increasing CHD risk.

Summary

In this chapter I have summarized a vast amount of research on diet, obesity, cholesterol and heart disease. It is an area that is fraught with speedbumps and potholes on the road to good health. The flawed dietary research is epitomized by individuals, such as Ancel Keys, who was guided not by profit, but by his bias against saturated fat, which interfered with his objectivity in realizing that a diet rich in fat and sugar can be blamed for much of modern society's poor health. Other work, specifically cholesterol research, has been guided to a great extent, by profit. The global hysteria to reduce serum cholesterol levels has been fuelled by the vast profits to food and drug companies which promise good health in exchange for using their products to lower cholesterol levels.

The findings summarized here indicate we have been misled to fear the cholesterol in our blood and the saturated fat in our food. Currently, millions of people around the world are treating their high cholesterol with lipid-lowering drugs, such as statins, with small benefits, if any, and serious side effects. It is time to test the blood coagulation hypothesis using a combination of a low carbohydrate diet, which by reducing blood sugar would reduce excess coagulation, and to assess anticoagulant approaches as more effective treatments than LDL lowering therapies.

David M. Diamond, PhD

Departments of Psychology, Molecular Pharmacology & Physiology, University of South Florida, Tampa, Florida, 33620

Reading List and On-Line Lectures

1. Atkins RC. Dr. Atkins' Diet Revolution. New York: Literary Guild; 1972.

2. Part 1 - Obesity and Fad Diets. In: Select Committee on Nutrition and Human Needs of the United States Senate Washington, D.C.: United States; 1973. p. 110.

3. A critique of low-carbohydrate ketogenic weight reduction regimens. A review of Dr. Atkins' diet revolution. JAMA 1973; 224:1415-1419.

4. Kirkpatrick CF, Bolick JP, Kris-Etherton PM *et al.* Review of current evidence and clinical recommendations on the effects of low-carbohydrate and very-low-carbohydrate (including ketogenic) diets for the management of body weight and other cardiometabolic risk factors: A scientific statement from the National Lipid Association Nutrition and Lifestyle Task Force. Journal of clinical lipidology 2019; 13:689-711 e681.

5. Brillat-Savarin JA. The Physiology of Taste (Translated by M.F.K. Fisher). The Heritage Press; 1949.

6. Banting W. Letter on Corpulence: Addressed to the Public. London: Banting; 1863.

7. Densmore E. The Natural Food of Man. New York: Stillman & Company; 1892.

8. Westman EC, Yancy WS, Jr., Humphreys M. Dietary treatment of diabetes mellitus in the pre-insulin era (1914-1922). Perspect Biol Med 2006; 49:77-83.

9. Pennington AW. Treatment of obesity: developments of the past 150 years. Am J Dig Dis 1954; 21:65-69.

10. PENNINGTON AW. A reorientation on obesity. N. Engl. J. Med 1953; 248:959-964.

11. Thorpe GL. Treating overweight patients. J Am Med Assoc 1957; 165:1361-1365.

12. Donaldson BF, Heyd CG. Strong Medicine. New York: Doubleday & Company; 1961.

13. Gordon ES, Goldberg M, Chosy GJ. A New Concept in the Treatment of Obesity. JAMA 1963; 186:50-60.

14. Keys A. Atherosclerosis: a problem in newer public health. J. Mt. Sinai Hosp. N. Y 1953; 20:118-139.

15. Green R. The Practice of Endocrinology. Philadelphia: Lippincott; 1951.

16. Yudkin J, Carey M. The treatment of obesity by the "highfat" diet. The inevitability of calories. *Lancet* 1960; 2:939-941.

17. Athinarayanan SJ, Adams RN, Hallberg SJ et al. Long-Term Effects of a Novel Continuous Remote Care Intervention Including Nutritional Ketosis for the Management of Type 2 Diabetes: A 2-Year Non-randomized Clinical Trial. Front Endocrinol (Lausanne) 2019; 10:348.

18. Rose GA, Thomson WB, Williams RT. Corn oil in treatment of ischaemic heart disease. Br. Med. J 1965; 1:1531-1533.

19. Ravnskov U, Dinicolantonio JJ, Harcombe Z et al. The questionable benefits of exchanging saturated fat with polyunsaturated fat. Mayo Clin. Proc 2014; 89:451-453.

20. Feinman RD, Pogozelski WK, Astrup A et al. Dietary carbohydrate restriction as the first approach in diabetes management: Critical review and evidence base. Nutrition 2015; 31:1-13.

21. The Lipid Research Clinics Coronary Primary Prevention Trial results. I. Reduction in incidence of coronary heart disease. JAMA 1984; 251:351-364.

22. Roberts WC. The underused miracle drugs: the statin drugs are to atherosclerosis what penicillin was to infectious disease. The American journal of cardiology 1996; 78:377-378.

23. Diamond DM, Ravnskov U. How statistical deception created the appearance that statins are safe and effective in primary and secondary prevention of cardiovascular disease. Expert Rev Clin Pharmacol 2015; 8:201-210.

24. Ridker PM, Danielson E, Fonseca FA et al. Rosuvastatin to prevent vascular events in men and women with elevated C-reactive protein. N Engl J Med 2008; 359:2195-2207.

25. Nutrition classics. Archives of Internal Medicine, Volume 64, October 1939: Angina pectoris in hereditary xanthomatosis. By Carl Muller. Nutr Rev 1987; 45:113-115.

26. Harlan WR, Graham JB, Estes EH. Familial Hypercholesterolemia – a Genetic and Metabolic Study. Medicine 1966; 45:77-&.

27. Mundal L, Sarancic M, Ose L *et al.* Mortality Among Patients With Familial Hypercholesterolemia: A Registry-Based Study in Norway, 1992-2010. Journal of the American Heart Association 2014; 3.

28. Brown MS, Goldstein JL. How LDL receptors influence cholesterol and atherosclerosis. Sci Am 1984; 251:58-66.

29. Ravnskov U, de Lorgeril M, Kendrick M, Diamond DM. Inborn coagulation factors are more important cardiovascular risk factors than high LDL-cholesterol in familial hypercholesterolemia. Med Hypotheses 2018; 121:60-63.

On-Line Lectures

David Diamond on Deception in Cholesterol Research: Separating Truth From Profitable Fiction. https://www.youtube.com/watch?v=inwfSkSGvQw

David Diamond, PhD. – A rigorous assessment of the myth that cholesterol causes heart disease. https://www.youtube.com/watch?v=SYlhG8_nZe0

David Diamond, PhD – Dietary Sense and Nonsense in the War on Saturated Fat. https://www.youtube.com/watch?v=J77Bweikiw8